Computers in Health Care

Kathryn J. Hannah   Marion J. Ball
Series Editors

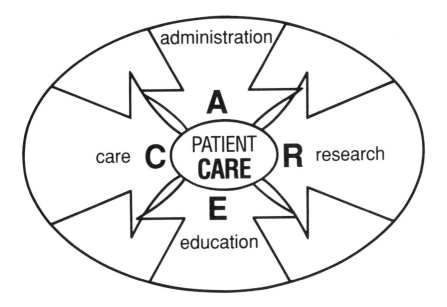

Computers in Health Care

Series Editors:
Kathryn J. Hannah   Marion J. Ball

Erica L. Drazen   Jane B. Metzger
Jami L. Ritter   Mark K. Schneider

Patient Care Information Systems

Successful Design and Implementation

With Contributions by
John P. Glaser   Samarjit Marwaha
William C. Reed   Jonathan M. Teich

With 33 Illustrations

Springer-Verlag

New York Berlin Heidelberg London Paris
Tokyo Hong Kong Barcelona Budapest

Erica L. Drazen
Arthur D. Little, Inc.
Acorn Park
Cambridge, MA 02140
USA

Jane B. Metzger
Arthur D. Little, Inc.
Acorn Park
Cambridge, MA 02140
USA

Jami L. Ritter
Arthur D. Little, Inc.
Acorn Park
Cambridge, MA 02140
USA

Mark K. Schneider
Arthur D. Little, Inc.
Acorn Park
Cambridge, MA 02140
USA

Library of Congress Cataloging-in-Publication Data
Patient care information systems: successful design and
   implementation / Erica L. Drazen . . . [et al.].
        p.   cm. — (Computers in health care)
   Includes bibliographical references and index.
   ISBN 0-387-94255-6. — ISBN 3-540-94255-6
      1. Information storage and retrieval systems — Medical care.
   2. Information storage and retrieval systems — Hospital. I. Drazen,
   Erica. II. Series: Computers in health care (New York, N.Y.)
      [DNLM: 1. Information Systems.   2. Delivery of Health Care —
   methods.   W 26.5 P298 1994]
   R858.P38   1994
   362.1′0285 — dc20   94-28728

Printed on acid-free paper.

Production coordinated by Chernow Editorial Services, Inc., and managed by Bill Imbornoni;
manufacturing supervised by Genieve Shaw.
Camera-ready copy provided by the authors.
Printed and bound by Edwards Brothers, Inc., Ann Arbor, MI.
Printed in the United States of America.

9 8 7 6 5 4 3 2 1

ISBN 0-387-94255-6 Springer-Verlag New York Berlin Heidelberg
ISBN 3-540-94255-6 Springer-Verlag Berlin Heidelberg New York

Series Preface

This series is intended for the rapidly increasing number of health care professionals who have rudimentary knowledge and experience in health care computing and are seeking opportunities to expand their horizons. It does not attempt to compete with the primers already on the market. Eminent international experts will edit, author, or contribute to each volume in order to provide comprehensive and current accounts of innovations and future trends in this quickly evolving field. Each book will be practical, easy to use, and well referenced.

Our aim is for the series to encompass all of the health professions by focusing on specific professions, such as nursing, in individual volumes. However, integrated computing systems are only one tool for improving communication among members of the health care team. Therefore, it is our hope that the series will stimulate professionals to explore additional means of fostering interdisplinary exchange.

This series springs from a professional collaboration that has grown over the years into a highly valued personal friendship. Our joint values put people first. If the Computers in Health Care series lets us share those values by helping health care professionals to communicate their ideas for the benefit of patients, then our efforts will have succeeded.

Kathryn J. Hannah
Marion J. Ball

Preface

Computer systems have been installed in hospitals and ambulatory care settings for decades. Over the years, the focus of investment has been shifting from patient accounting and billing systems to systems for handling data from clinical and administrative services (pharmacy, laboratory, admitting). The most recent advance is toward development and use of systems that support the delivery of patient care by aggregating relevant information from different sources and providing access to that information in a form that supports health care providers in making decisions about a patient's care.

Why has it taken so long for computers to be used in delivery of patient care — *the* primary business of health care institutions? Why has interest in these systems suddenly escalated? Several different explanations have been offered. One view is that physicians have resisted computer support, and that resistance is just beginning to break down as more computer literate staff join the work force. As we will explain in Chapter 2, there is little evidence to support this theory. In fact, studies over the last two decades have documented positive attitudes toward computers among physicians and nurses. We think that physicians and nurses have always *wanted* useful computer support, and now they are *demanding* it.

Lack of appropriate technology is another often-cited barrier to the implementation of patient care computers. However, the Institute of Medicine's report on the computer-based patient record concluded that the technology to support computer-based records is available.(1) As some of the references in later chapters will document, patient care information systems were developed and successfully implemented using the technology available in the 1960s and 1970s. Many of these systems are still in use today.

Although technological advances have significantly increased the number of options for display formats, input and output devices, and back-up and security systems, the basic technology to create a useful information system for health care has existed for some time. Advances in information and communications standards and the "open systems" movement have enabled institutions to move toward patient care information systems without abandoning all of their current computer investment. As we will discuss in Chapter 4, we believe that technological advances will enhance the solutions available, but that the most critical element of a patient care information system is in the logic, screen flow, and design of the end-user support. This was the "secret to success" of some of the earliest patient care information systems and the missing element of many unsuccessful systems today.

Another theory about the evolution of patient care computing is that health care institutions have made computer investments in response to external pressures. Hospitals first acquired computer systems during the era when payment for care was based on cost reimbursement. At that time, two critical issues for the hospital were accounting for costs (to justify charges for the following year) and sending bills out quickly (to manage cash flow). Patient billing was the first application to be automated, and then revenue-producing departments were automated to capture charges for services. Later, automation was applied to improve operational efficiency and lower costs in laboratory, pharmacy, and radiology departments. Since many of these services faced outside competition, there was pressure to control costs and provide good service.

Currently, the demands on the health care delivery system are to lower costs and to be accountable for outcomes over a continuum of care. As we will discuss in Chapter 1, there is an abundance of evidence that computer support can make significant contributions to patient management. Under prospective payment, capitation, or fixed-fee schedules, institutions must continually try to lower costs and improve services to remain competitive. Most of the day-to-day resource consumption that drives operating costs is determined by physicians and nurses when they develop plans of care and order tests and treatments. Health care delivery institutions need to help these users make cost-effective decisions, provide managers with the information they need to monitor access to and outcomes of care, and improve the process of care delivery.

As we move to deliver care within an integrated, community-based delivery system, the need for information and the difficulty in accessing information increase simultaneously. It is impossible to provide seamless access to care without also providing seamless access to information; patients will not be directed to the most appropriate location of care unless relevant information about the patient can be directed there also. *We believe these pressures are the major forces behind the current interest in patient care computer systems.*

When looking toward the future, three things seem clear.

- The need for patient care information systems will only increase over time.
- Success in implementing patient care systems will be critical to building viable integrated care delivery systems.

- Supporting patient care with information systems will require a huge investment of capital, management attention, and staff time.

How much progress have we made in implementing patient care systems, and what have we learned?

National market data from 3,000 hospitals indicate that hospitals spent $5.5B in information systems in 1990.(2) Investments in systems for clinical departments are increasing at a rate of 20 to 40 percent per year. The penetration of patient care information systems is so small that they have not been tracked in national surveys. However, in a 1992 survey of chief executive officers of 27 hospitals and multihospital systems, most stated that their long-term vision is to have an integrated information system containing all clinical and financial information.(2) Clearly, we are not there yet.

In a 1993 survey, hospital CEOs rated their information position on a scale of 1 to 5, where 1 was not prepared and 5 was completely prepared. CEOs rated their preparedness for the following as a 3: for meeting information requirements for JCAHO initiatives on clinical quality, TQM/CQI initiatives, networking with physician practices, clinical outcomes management, collaboration with other hospitals, patient-centered care initiatives, EDI and computerized patient records, and managed care.(3) Unfortunately, this list almost completely overlaps the list of initiatives that are most critical to success within the new health care delivery environment. Perhaps even more alarming (at least for current CIOs) is that 21 percent of the CEOs felt their current CIOs would not be capable of implementing necessary changes in information support, and 53 percent of CEOs admitted *they did not know* if their CIOs were capable of leading them into the future.

There are many alternative uses for the billions of dollars that will need to be invested in information systems. It is imperative that investment decisions be made wisely and that the capabilities acquired provide real value in patient care and institutional management. Without question, many system developers, health care institutions, and system vendors have learned valuable lessons about how to design, develop, implement, and use patient care computer systems. However, much of this knowledge is inaccessible because it has never been published or because the only publications have been in conference proceedings, which are typically not indexed, not readily available in libraries, and often out of print. In this book, we have attempted to summarize and synthesize lessons learned from the past so they can provide a basis for future progress.

There are several potential impediments to using past experience to guide the future design, selection, and use of patient care information systems. One problem relates to the fact that there is no one "patient care information system." Available systems differ in the capabilities they offer (the type of information that is available), in the user interface (e.g., ease of use, method of data entry), and in the technical performance of the system (e.g., response time and down time). Products are also continually evolving. Because most studies only report on the experience with one system at one point in time, it is difficult to separate out effects related to the particular system being studied from the effects of computer systems in general.

The use of existing systems also differs. The computers may be used directly by physicians and nurses, nurses or clerical staff may transcribe physicians' orders into the system, and these same staff may use the system to retrieve results for physicians. Use may be either voluntary or mandatory. Mandatory use typically implies not only that is there a directive to use the system, but also that alternative manual methods for obtaining information are no longer available. Most studies are conducted in only one institution, with computer systems that duplicate or replace some part of the paper medical record with automation. It is, therefore, difficult to generalize about use of computers across different settings with different approaches to using the system.

Despite these limitations, to accelerate the rate of progress we as a nation are making in the use of patient care computers, we need to mine all the value we can from past experience. It is our hope that this volume will be a significant contribution toward advancing our understanding of best practices for providing information support to patient care.

What is a patient care information system? There is no standard definition, but in the broadest sense, the system will provide access to all of the information needed to effectively care for a patient. As shown in Figure P-1, there are three main categories of patient care information — information related to the patient; information that is specific for each institution; and information relative to the professional domain of each user. Today's patient care information systems contain a subset of these data. Items with a bullet on Figure P–1 are available in many patient care information systems today. Items with an arrow are not being used except in a few test sites. The remaining elements are found in some commercial products today and are likely to be found in advanced patient care information systems developed by institutions themselves.

There are several other elements of a good patient care information system:

- At a minimum, all data are stored at a patient level and retrievable in an integrated form for any patient.
- A comprehensive patient care information system is linked to a communication system to ensure that information is available to all relevant care givers. The system does *not* require caregivers to perform administrative functions — all administrative data are generated as a by-product of care delivery.

This book is focused on meeting the information needs of direct care givers. Much of the discussion, and most of the research, has focused on

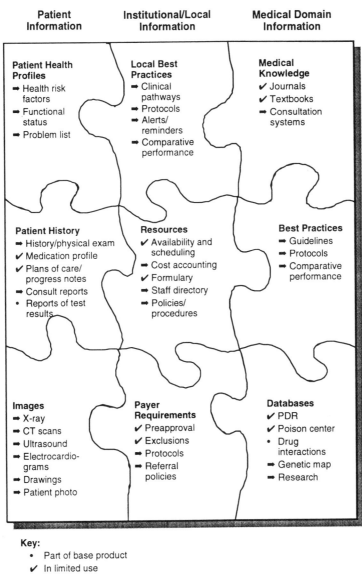

| Patient Information | Institutional/Local Information | Medical Domain Information |

Patient Health Profiles
→ Health risk factors
→ Functional status
→ Problem list

Local Best Practices
→ Clinical pathways
→ Protocols
→ Alerts/ reminders
→ Comparative performance

Medical Knowledge
✔ Journals
✔ Textbooks
→ Consultation systems

Patient History
→ History/physical exam
✔ Medication profile
✔ Plans of care/ progress notes
→ Consult reports
• Reports of test results

Resources
✔ Availability and scheduling
→ Cost accounting
✔ Formulary
→ Staff directory
→ Policies/ procedures

Best Practices
→ Guidelines
→ Protocols
→ Comparative performance

Images
→ X-ray
→ CT scans
→ Ultrasound
→ Electrocardio- grams
→ Drawings
→ Patient photo

Payer Requirements
✔ Preapproval
✔ Exclusions
→ Protocols
→ Referral policies

Databases
✔ PDR
✔ Poison center
• Drug interactions
→ Genetic map
→ Research

Key:
• Part of base product
✔ In limited use
→ Emerging

Figure P-1. Elements of a Comprehensive Patient Care Information System

computer use by physicians both because physicians' decisions affect so much of the cost of care delivery and because this group has traditionally not used computer systems. We have also included information about patient care information support within nursing. However, a very comprehensive review of information requirements to support nursing has been published(4) and comprehensive references in the area of nursing informatics are available.(5,6) We have not duplicated these efforts.

One of our conclusions about information support for patient care is that the "end-user views" will need to be tailored for different users. This does not mean that each set of users will have their own system. In fact, we think that the concept of specialized nursing systems, physical therapy systems, etc., is fundamentally flawed. What is needed is one patient care information system with end-user support tailored to the needs of specific groups of providers. We expect that the experience gained in supporting nurses and physicians will provide excellent guidance on how to support the needs of all those who will be providing patient care in the future (including patients themselves).

The objective of this book is to put the knowledge that we have gained to work. We have assembled information on successful design, selection, and implementation of patient care computer systems from available sources and summarized it to create one resource book. We have tried to cover the selected topics comprehensively; as part of this effort we performed traditional literature searches and reviewed conference proceedings. We have also included information gained during our years of consulting on patient care information systems; and we asked several colleagues, who are on the leading edge of patient care computing in health care delivery settings, to share their experiences from the "front lines."

There is mounting evidence that computer systems not only provide value in health care delivery but also that they may be essential to effective implementation of protocols, to ensure compliance with guidelines, and to provide a continuum of patient care. This experience is reviewed in Chapter 1. However, to put computer tools to work, they must be accepted by physicians, nurses, and other care givers. In Chapter 2 we review experiences with physicians' and nurses' acceptance of computers and dispel some prevailing myths.

Chapter 3 presents case studies of the acceptance and impact of stand-alone departmental systems and an integrated patient care information system. The case studies are based on multisite trials. We feel that both the findings of the studies and the lessons learned about evaluating systems provide useful information for future planning.

In Chapter 4 we review the lessons learned in design of system support for physicians and nurses — features and functions that contributed to success and to failure in the past. This information will be useful to designers of future systems and also to institutions who are evaluating alternative systems for purchase.

Chapter 5 outlines approaches to developing a plan for patient care information systems, and in Chapter 6 we discuss success approaches and the required organization for executing these plans. Chapter 7 takes a future orientation, and we discuss the forces that are driving change in patient care information needs, the user roles that will be supported in the future, and the technologies that will be used.

A Future Scenario

Because we are so far from reaching our ideal of a patient care information system, we will close with a future scenario that was adopted from an information systems plan developed by a health care system.(7)

It is a pleasant Sunday afternoon in suburban anywhere, in the spring of 1999. Mary Smith, who just celebrated her ninetieth birthday, is worried. She just has not been feeling right — slightly dizzy, short of breath, and she cannot keep food down. Mary is trying to decide if she should call her daughter to take her to the urgent care center; she certainly does not want to bother her nice, new, young doctor with her complaints. Mary finally decides to do something; she walks over to the health access terminal in her den and logs on. She quickly enters her symptoms, responds to a few questions, and then reads a return message: "Mary, the symptoms you describe may require treatment. While there is no cause for alarm, you should go to Saint Vincent's urgent care center this afternoon. We will notify Dr. Jones, who is covering for your group. He will be expecting to see you. If you need directions to the center, or help with transportation, please press the HELP key or call 465-7895."

Meanwhile, Dr. Jones, who is traveling along the highway, hears his pager beep. A voice message gives him a summary of the situation and the advice given to Mary. Dr. Jones pulls over; through a modem on his cellular phone, he connects to the health network. From his list of action items, he selects "view Mary Smith" and reviews a summary of Mary's interaction with her health access terminal, and her "quick view" health record that contains a problem list, current medications, and summary of recent visits. He notes that Mary recently saw a specialist at City Hospital for her asthma and is on a new medication. Dr. Jones clicks his computer pointer on that medication and is linked into the Physicians' Desk Reference. He reviews the latest information on potential side effects. Dr. Jones also makes a mental note of the health screening reminder that Mary is overdue for a tetanus shot. He will make sure that this is taken care of when he sees Mary.

At Saint Vincent's, Mary's name appears on the urgent care unit's "expect log." There is a note on the log that Dr. Jones has reviewed Mary's record and that his preference is to be notified as soon as the patient arrives. (The computer will do this automatically.) If Mary does not come into the unit within 2 hours, the patient advocate in the unit will call her at home.

Based on the symptoms Mary entered on her health access terminal, the clinic's computer system has retrieved a suggested protocol for treating Mary on arrival and a schedule for testing has been developed. Thirty minutes later Mary arrives and is greeted by name by the receptionist — who recognizes her from her picture on the "expect log" computer screen. Mary is taken directly into a room; the nurse examines Mary and takes her blood pressure. (The results are automatically transmitted to update Mary's record.) The nurse reviews the computer-generated plan of care for Mary on a screen in the exam room and through the voice command "Agree" automatically sends orders for tests to the appropriate departments. Dr. Jones is beeped again; he calls to say he is on his way in. The call is routed to Mary's room, where her care provider picks up the call on a wireless receiver in her name badge. Dr. Jones tells Mary he will see her soon. Mary is feeling much better already.

Erica L. Drazen

References

1. Dick RS and Steen EB. The computer-based patient record: an essential technology for health care. Washington, DC: National Academy Press, 1991.
2. Dorenfest SI. Hospital information systems: the state of the art. Chicago: Sheldon Dorenfest Associates Limited, 1992.
3. Hard R. The real thing: future information needs will require "true" hospital CIOs. Hospitals, February 20, 1993; pp. 36–40.
4. Zielstorff R, Hudgings C, Grobe, S. Next generation nursing information systems. Washington, DC: American Nurses Publishers, 1993.
5. Ball MJ, Hannah KJ, Jelger UG, Peterson H. Nursing informatics, where caring and technology meet. New York: Springer-Verlag, 1988.
6. Hannah KJ, Ball MJ, Edwards MJA. Introduction to nursing informatics. New York: Springer-Verlag, 1993.
7. Daughters of Charity National Health System. Report on DCNHS Task Force on Information Needs. 1993.

Acknowledgments

The heritage of this book lies in Arthur D. Little's information systems practice over the last 25 years. A large number of groups and individuals are responsible for the collective experience it represents:

- Current and former colleagues at Arthur D. Little, Inc., who contributed creative energy, problem-solving skills, and insights.
- Clients in health care institutions, the vendor industry, and Government who provided IS consulting and research assignments that have taken us into many health care environments and given us opportunities to study and witness the potential and pitfalls of information support to patient care and to learn practical lessons about how to achieve the full potential.
- Innumerable current and prospective users of patient care information systems – physicians, nurses, business managers, and others – who allowed us to observe their work environment and shared their experiences and thoughts about prerequisites for success.

We are indebted to them all. Some specific contributors deserve special mention.

Chapters 2 and 3 grew out of Erica Drazen's thesis research. Thanks are due to a thesis committee of Heather Palmer and John Orav from the Harvard School of Public Health, Warner Slack of the Center for Clinical Computing and the Harvard Medical School, and Judith Hall from Northeastern University. They patiently guided the thinking for the research design and the analysis of the multi-center trial of patient care computers that forms the basis of the case studies in Chapter 3 and the research review in Chapter 2. The officials and staff members within the Department of Defense, and in particular CAPT Paul Tibbits, sponsored the questionnaire surveys of physicians and nurses reported in Chapter 3. Dr. Tibbits welcomed the opportunity to incorporate academic rigor into the DoD evaluation process, maintained the momentum of the project, and also advocated sharing results of their experience.

Our sometimes clients, always colleagues, on the "front lines," who agreed to coauthor chapters were invaluable in ensuring that this book maintained a practical bent.

John Glaser, whom we miss as a fellow staff member but enjoy as a client, has given us the opportunity to watch and help in building the patient care information system at the Brigham and Women's Hospital and coauthored Chapter 6. By working with Jonathan Teich also at the Brigham, we have become much smarter about how to design systems physicians will willingly use. His help on Chapter 4 was invaluable, and we believe the examples from the Brigham system will make the design concepts real for readers.

Bill Reed gave us an invaluable opportunity to participate in planning for information systems to support a truly integrated system of care. We appreciate Bill's help in writing Chapter 5.

Sam Marwaha has recently decided to make health care a focus of his information systems practice at Arthur D. Little. We welcome his expertise on our projects, as well as his assistance in predicting the future in Chapter 7. Sam and others have helped us incorporate the role environment approach, discussed in Chapters 6 and 7, into our practice. Stephen Kramer, Halen Armian-Hawley, and Barbara Perron all contributed to developing the new health care roles — direct care and business roles — in Chapter 7. Tony Christy assisted by programming the demonstration version of the health care role environment for the Primary Care Manager/Gatekeeper. Barbara Perron and David Stasior helped us get the clinical details correct.

We never would have completed this book without technical support from Barbara Kendall, Denise Smith, and Barbara Wyse. They helped with the editing, production, and sheparding of the (many) drafts from start to finish. Joanne Frate was a wizard at tracking down the obscure references we needed for many chapters. Research assistance for Chapters 6 and 7 was also provided by Joanne Adamowicz and Beverly Colby. Celia Doremus, from our marketing department, assisted in our early discussions with Springer when this book was merely a concept. Long after our writing is complete, Celia's work will continue as she endeavors to ensure this book reaches you, our readers.

Our editors at Springer, in particular Andrea Seils, had the ideal balance of encouragement, insistence, and patience to keep us going, yet they understood that we also all have "real" jobs and "real" clients with urgent problems that require our attention.

Finally, we need to acknowledge the patience of our families. The constant travel of consulting is hard on families, but combining that with the large amount of after-hours and weekend work required to write a book *truly requires* understanding.

We hope our readers will learn as much from reading the end product as we learned from creating it. Best wishes on your journey to implement patient care information systems that help you achieve your institutional objectives.

Contents

Contributors

Erica L. Drazen
Arthur D. Little, Inc.
Acorn Park
Cambridge, MA 02140

John P. Glaser
Information Systems
Brigham and Women's Hospital
Boston, MA 02115

Samarjit Marwaha
Arthur D. Little, Inc.
Acorn Park
Cambridge, MA 02140

Jane B. Metzger
Arthur D. Little, Inc.
Acorn Park
Cambridge, MA 02140

William C. Reed
Geisinger Health System
100 North Academy Avenue
Danville, PA 17822-3011

Dr. Jami Ritter
Arthur D. Little, Inc.
Acorn Park
Cambridge, MA 02140

Mark K. Schneider
Arthur D. Little, Inc.
Acorn Park
Cambridge, MA 02140

Jonathan M. Teich
Center for Applied Medical
    Information Systems
Brigham and Women's Hospital
Boston, MA 02115

1
The Potential Contributions of Patient Care Information Systems

Jane B. Metzger

The current interest in patient care information systems stems from two basic convictions:

- We are paying a high cost in decreased efficiency and quality by managing patient care relying on paper-based records and separate computer systems that capture one type of clinical or administrative information.
- Patient care information systems have the potential to overcome current breakdowns and inefficiencies in patient information processes and to leverage information in ways that were never possible before.

This chapter reviews some of the evidence that supports these two convictions.

The Cost of the Status Quo

Since their conception, the principal motivation for implementing patient care information systems is that current information management practices do not permit us to provide health care efficiently and with consistently high quality. We expend a significant portion of available health care resources on creating, storing, and retrieving patient information in labor-intensive, redundant, and often ineffective efforts to document care and to provide a reliable information resource for physicians, nurses, and other direct care providers. With administrative costs accounting for nearly 25 percent of hospital budgets in the United States, trimming administrative overhead is an obvious tactic for cost containment.(1)

Despite our current investment in patient information, physicians and other direct care providers are severely hampered in providing timely, appropriate, and efficient health care to their patients because they often lack the information they need or they spend more time searching for and assembling information than in their primary mission–taking care of patients. Anyone who works in direct care or who has reviewed or worked with medical records is aware of these deficiencies, and considerable evidence has been accumulated to use in describing and quantifying this problem. This section reviews some of this evidence and the related impacts on the quality and efficiency of health care.

Paper Medical Records

Paper medical records remain the legal, official record of patient care. Although in some health care organizations computer-generated information comprises part of the medical record, file folders full of slips of paper and massive file rooms are still the norm today. Some physicians, nurses, and other care professionals can obtain some of the patient information they need (i.e., most likely laboratory and possibly radiology results) from computer terminals located in patient care areas, but most health care providers still rely on paper medical records as the primary source of patient information. Many aspects of the processes whereby records are created and maintained make them unwieldy (and often bulky), unreliable (completeness and accuracy), unavailable (because they have been misfiled, lost/borrowed, or are in transit), and difficult to use.

Much of the information in medical records is handwritten, especially patient problem lists, documentation of history and physical, and encounter notes in outpatient records and order sheets and progress notes in inpatient records. One of the drawbacks of handwritten documentation is obviously illegibility. This is less of a problem for the physician or nurse who originally penned the text, but can be extremely difficult for others who must devote extra time to the task of reading it and may not end up with the information they need. In one report concerning a research study based on emergency department notes, physicians had to be asked to dictate their notes for transcription because it was so difficult to obtain the information needed for the study from the handwritten documentation.(2)

When documentation is handwritten, it tends to be free form and, though guided in some cases by headings on preprinted forms, not necessarily complete. In one review of outpatient records at five hospitals, neither the problem nor the treatment was adequately described in encounter notes 10 percent of the time, and general medical information useful for preventive medicine was lacking in 27 to 60 percent of the records.(3) When verbatim transcripts of outpatient visits were compared with information recorded in medical records in another study, the chief complaint was recorded in the record 92 percent of the time, information relating to the present illness was provided 71 percent of the time, but other medical history discussed during the encounter was recorded only 29 percent of the time.(4)

Because medical nomenclature is not standardized, it is difficult to ensure that the user of a medical record draws the interpretation from the documentation that the author intended. In one review of problem lists in approximately 1,500 outpatient medical records, hypertension was recorded a total of 103 ways (including misspellings).(5)

Many events must occur for all of the documentation for a particular patient to end up filed in the appropriate medical record:

- Record elements must contain appropriate (and legible) patient-identifying information.
- They have to emerge from the department or clinical area in which they were created enroute to the medical record room.
- They must be received in the location where the patient's medical record is maintained.
- They need to be filed in the correct medical record (or eventually meet up with the medical record if it happens to be signed out at the time).

With so many opportunities for things to go awry, it is not surprising that they do, especially when large numbers of patients, records, and slips of paper are involved.

We audited the outpatient medical records in ambulatory care settings in three hospitals that maintain centralized records and discovered:

- In one site, nearly 8,000 loose record elements could not be filed because the patient's medical record had not been located; several hundred of these lacked any patient identification.
- In another site, 20 percent of randomly selected records contained at least one record element with a different name or patient number than on the record jacket.
- In all three study sites, each randomly selected record had an average of two record elements lacking the patient number and two or three containing no patient identification whatsoever.(6)

Each unfiled or possibly misfiled record element presumably represented a deficiency (or potential deficiency) in some other patient's medical record.

Record elements are generally filed by source (e.g., laboratory results slips together) and (roughly) by time. One practicing physician has characterized typical office records as "a loose leaf jumble . . . folders thickly packed with sheets of different sizes, designs and colors with life-and-death findings mixed indiscriminately with unsorted normal data."(7)

For inpatients, the number of pages in a patient's chart accumulates rapidly. In one large teaching hospital, 130 different kinds of information were identified in paper records for discharged patients; the average record size was 109 pages.

Record sizes for inpatients on different medical services ranged from 197 pages (Shock Trauma) to 29 pages (Newborn).(8) The same practicing physician cited earlier has characterized the typical inpatient record as a "disorganized encyclopedia," unable to provide complete or completely legible information, not sorted for relevance, and with an "unmanageable form [of] divisions, crumpled tabs, three-ring notebook with clips and loose papers."(7)

Direct Care Processes

Hospitals and large ambulatory care centers have elaborate and costly processes in place to pull medical records and make them available in the locations where physicians and other providers need the information. Because of timing (especially for walk-in and emergency patients) and the difficulty of locating (and often delivering) records, however, many patients end up being seen without a medical record. Data from numerous different published reports provide insight into the magnitude of this problem:

- In a series of studies in large outpatient clinics with centralized patient records (and no patient information available via computer), we found that the percentage of patients seen without a medical record ranged from 6 to 18 percent.(6)
- In one review of record availability at five hospitals, as many as 30 percent of the patients in an individual clinic session were seen without a medical record, and no past medical data was available for 11 percent of all of the patients in the sample.(3)
- Analysis of outpatient record availability in another hospital documented that records were unavailable in 15 percent of the ambulatory encounters.(9)

Medical records are typically maintained in each care setting. Patients who obtain care in multiple organizations or settings have fragmented, partial documentation of their medical history in a number of different records. Many patients see physicians in a number of different office practice settings, where separate medical records are maintained. Even in hospital-based ambulatory clinics where official medical records are maintained centrally, many physicians maintain duplicate office records because of the problems in reliably accessing official medical records. Physicians in any one setting who consult locally maintained medical records obviously are severely limited in their ability to access complete information about the patients under their care. This problem will greatly increase if we attempt to create integrated care delivery systems without the information infrastructure to support seamless access to patient information.

Not every patient interaction requires extensive patient information from a medical record, and the real significance of missing or incomplete records varies from one case to another. However, the issue of *missing* information necessary to manage the case at hand has been explored in several studies in which physicians themselves have identified the lack of needed information:

- For a sample of patients in multiple large primary and specialty outpatient clinics in each of three different hospitals, physicians and other providers (such as physician's assistants) reported that information deemed necessary was missing 18 to 20 percent of the time.(6)
- In another study involving a large number of patients seen in clinics in seven hospitals and three free-standing ambulatory care centers, physicians reported that information was missing for 15.2 percent of the patients seen during the study period.(10)
- Physicians in another study reported the following rates of missing information in outpatient records in five different hospitals: 17, 22, 25, 6, and 23 percent of encounters.(3)

One consequence of missing information can be repeat diagnostic tests and procedures. During some of our research in large ambulatory care clinics in three hospitals, physicians reported that they ordered a repeat test or consult for 3 to 5 percent of all patients due to missing information and had to schedule an additional visit as a result for 2 to 4 percent of their patients (presumably to accomplish follow-up on the results of the repeated testing or consult).(6)

Another consequence of missing information can be delays. One study in a teaching hospital detected, quantified, and ascribed causes of unnecessary delays in inpatient stays. Over a 6-month period, 30 percent of patients experienced delays averaging 2.9 days. For 3.8 percent of patients, a delay involved failure to obtain test results within a standard turnaround time, and 11.6 percent experienced a delay due to test scheduling (average length of delay for each of these two causes was 1.74 days).(11)

Many of the processes in health care delivery involve numerous steps, many different players, and pieces of paper traveling among departments via internal distribution. This presents numerous opportunities for needed information to be lost or delayed. One decision analysis of the process for follow-up of positive test results identified eight possible decision nodes where standards of practice permitted performance evaluation; 52 percent of the cases reviewed failed to meet standards at one or more of these nodes, and many of the deviations represented a breakdown in an information process (e.g., test result not in chart) or a failure to respond to information.(12) Another analysis of routine clinical processes revealed that failure rates could be as high as 33 percent. For the processes of obtaining mammograms and referrals, identified process improvements all involved better, more reliable communication of information or the ability to track service completion.(13)

Another consequence of delayed or missing information can be a delay in treatment. In the Harvard study of medical injury and malpractice in the State of New York, 10.3 percent of physician errors leading to adverse events in hospitalized patients resulted from failure to act upon results of tests or findings and 9.4 percent resulted from an avoidable delay in diagnosis.(14) This research did not explore the specific contribution of information process breakdowns. In our unpublished research on the potential contributions of patient care information systems to quality of care, we had an opportunity to review case summaries for medical malpractice claims. We found it easy to identify cases where an information process breakdown such as lack of follow-up of abnormal diagnostic results, especially radiology results, was a root cause of (or major contributor to) the patient injury claimed.

For some types of critical patient information, elaborate mechanisms are devised to ensure that potentially life-threatening conditions are responded to immediately. One example is critical value reporting for laboratory test results. Standard procedure is typically to telephone the physician's office and/or the inpatient unit to which the patient is assigned. In one study of critical value reporting, only 9.5 percent of the laboratory critical values tracked were telephoned to the patient's inpatient unit and only 15 percent of the charts for patients with a critical value contained documentation that a physician or nurse had received notification.(15)

In addition to errors of omission in care delivery, breakdowns in information processes can result in errors of commission. It has been estimated that 3 to 5 percent of admissions to hospitals are primarily for a drug reaction, 18 to 30 percent of hospitalized patients have a drug reaction, and 70 to 80 percent are potentially avoidable.(16) In one study of hospitalized adults, 0.9 percent of hospital days had a drug-related adverse event, 56 percent of which were judged to be preventable.(17)

Efficiency of Care Providers

Estimates of total physician and nurse time devoted to information handling range as high as 30 to 40 percent.(18,19) Nearly three decades ago Jydstrup and Gross estimated the total time devoted to information handling in an entire institution; they concluded that information handling accounted for nearly 24 percent of operating costs (average for three hospitals), with 25 percent of available personnel time on nursing units devoted to information handling.(20) No comparable hospital-wide estimates have been compiled from detailed observations of current practices and processes. The numbers would undoubtedly be much higher as the combined result of the increasing information intensity of medical practice in the intervening 30 years and all of the current information-based processes focused on utilization review and quality assurance.

One factor that contributes to time spent in information-related tasks is the form of the paper medical record, which makes it difficult for physicians and other care providers to obtain the information they need, particularly when the question involves patient status over a period of time as in,

Has this patient's weight been changing? or

What is the highest blood pressure recorded?

Researchers in one study of medical record formats asked physicians to review traditionally organized medical records for the information to answer these common questions. Reviewing outpatient records containing data from seven to 15 encounters (average record size of 45 pages) took 26.8 seconds on average for the first question and 57.6 seconds for the second question; reviewing records for inpatients after seven to 15 days in the hospital (average record size of 75 pages) took 36.6 and 37.4 seconds, respectively.(21)

It is not difficult to see how these times could add up when the physician needs to answer a series of information questions for an individual patient and/or is dealing with many patients. In one analysis of the cost justification for clinical applications and distributed workstations in an academic medical center, the authors concluded that only a 4 percent savings in time (20 minutes per day) for professional staff was required to break even on the investment in providing user access to the system.(22)

A frustrated practicing physician (the same one cited previously) has provided the following description of how the rounding physician assembles information for an inpatient (even when some diagnostic results are available from a computer terminal at the nursing station):

1. Find the "heat sheet" to determine the temperature and vital signs.
2. Locate the "Medex" to check on medications and when these were administered.
3. Find the nurses' notes or the nurse caring for that patient.
4. Find the record and convince others trying to use it that you need it.
5. Rummage through the record, with its crumpled tabs, for lab data, pathology reports, X-ray reports, and consultation notes (which are usually late and often misfiled).
6. Check the orders to see what has been ordered by the house staff.
7. Call up those laboratory and radiology results that are available by computer; call the laboratory directly for those that are not.
8. Go to the radiology department and begin another search for films and reports.
9. Finally, see the patient and family.(7)

One typical step omitted from this description is the practice of transcribing summary notes regarding significant facts or findings derived from these various, fragmented sources on an index card for future reference.

Several detailed time studies provide insight into the time that both physicians and nurses devote to seeking and creating paper-based patient information.

Work sampling studies on inpatient units in three hospitals yielded the following results for nursing time allocated to information tasks:

- Nursing unit personnel (nurses, nursing assistants, and ward clerks) spent 23 to 32 percent of total available time on clerical tasks such as reading and writing in patient charts, filling out test requisitions, and preparing administrative reports.
- Nurses spent 48 to 54 percent of their time in the combined activities of communication, end-of-shift report/conference, and clerical tasks.(6)

Most of the studies of physician time devoted to inpatient care have involved house staff at teaching hospitals. One time-motion study of Internal Medicine interns on call from 10 am to 8 pm in a large academic medical center indicated that nearly half of their time was devoted to information gathering and documentation. They spent 20 percent of their time talking person to person (50 percent of the time discussing a particular patient, 20 percent talking to patients, and 20 percent to other interns at changeover). Activities such as reading patient charts, laboratory results, and textbooks accounted for 12 percent of their time, while note writing consumed an additional 8 percent, and talking on the telephone 8 percent. Examining patients and staff rounds accounted for only 6 and 5 percent of their time, respectively.(23)

Another time study of Internal Medicine house staff on duty at night in two hospitals also showed that they spent considerable time charting. Documenting a new patient's history and physical examination took interns from 21 to 44 minutes per patient and residents from 17 to 26 minutes. (The authors noted that taking the history and performing the physical examination took less time than charting the results.)(24)

Studies of physician time in ambulatory care are more difficult to accomplish because of the need for patient privacy, and there are only a few data points. In one study of a small number of encounters, physicians spent a large portion of their total patient time (35 to 48 percent) interacting with the chart or performing other paperwork.(25) A work sampling study of residents and interns in a general medicine clinic provided similar results: during patient visits they spent 37.8 percent of their time charting, 5.3 percent consulting, 55.2 percent with the patient, and 1.7 percent in miscellaneous activities.(26)

When physicians cannot find the information they need, they typically spend considerable time attempting to locate it via telephone or (as mentioned in the process description preceding) perhaps by even going to another area or department. In our studies in outpatient clinics, physicians reported that they spent time looking for missing information during 10 to 13 percent of their patient encounters (and were unsuccessful in locating the needed information for 2 to 7 percent of their patients).(6)

In another study in an academic medical center, physicians estimated that they called the Radiology Department to obtain results for 28 to 32 percent of the radiology procedures they ordered for outpatients and inpatients, respectively, and went to the Radiology Department themselves (often a considerable distance) in search of reports and images for 32 percent of outpatient procedures and 60 percent of inpatient procedures. When these estimates were combined with conservative times per telephone call and visit to Radiology, it appeared that these physicians were devoting substantial time each day in seeking out just this one type of patient information.(27) Today's concept of the ultimate patient care information system would provide distributed access to both reports *and* images and potentially eliminate all such telephone calls and visits.

Evidence of Improvements Available from Patient Care Information Systems

Information about the potential benefits of patient care information systems has always been important in justifying the investment. Luckily, considerable research has produced evidence of quantified improvements in efficiency and quality achieved with real systems in real health care organizations, as well as many anecdotal reports describing the changes introduced. The following sections summarize this accumulated experience, first the benefits of improved access to information in outpatient and inpatient care, then the potential value-added through decision support capabilities, the benefits to research and practice improvement, and then the evidence concerning physicians as direct users of patient care information systems.

Improved Information Access–Ambulatory Care

One of the most immediate impacts of electronic access to patient information is the increased reliability of obtaining information. Once the information needed by providers is available online or in printed summaries of pertinent information from a clinical or ambulatory medical record system, system reliability and the availability of system access become the only limiting factors. In one report concerning the implementation of COSTAR, the system was available to provide needed information 99.05 percent of the time, an improvement over the previous 72 percent paper medical record availability.(28) In another early report concerning the same system in another setting, paper medical records were available 28 or 33 percent of the time (two measurements), and the system reliability was 98 percent.(29) [A number of existing automated ambulatory record systems provide access to pertinent patient information in a summary printed in advance of each scheduled patient encounter.(25,30-32)]

Providers do not need access to all historical information for every patient encounter. We studied the impact of a hospital-wide system that provided access to laboratory and radiology services, outpatient medications, and appointment history on physicians' access to patient information that *they felt was needed* for each patient encounter. The percentage of visits for which all needed information was available was 85 percent before the system was installed and increased to 95 percent afterwards.(10)

In addition to more reliable access, computer-stored information can be arranged and formatted so that physicians and other users can find what they need much more quickly. The paper medical record has a fixed format determined by the sequence and organization of the original recording of the information, whereas a patient care system can provide virtually unlimited options for sequencing, formatting, and combining different types of data into a single display.(33) This improved organization of information can greatly reduce the time physicians and other providers need to invest in assembling patient information for each patient encounter. One study showed that a fixed flowsheet format for patient information enables providers to obtain information in approximately 25 percent of the time that it takes to obtain information from a traditional paper record.(21) (Design features that provide added value by enhancing the ease of obtaining information are discussed in Chapter 4.)

Several studies have documented time savings for physicians and nurses in outpatient practice. In one early report from the initial COSTAR site(28):

- Nurses spent 3.5 minutes obtaining current medications from paper records, and 1.25 minutes from COSTAR.
- Assembling information to determine the last date and result of each test on a testing protocol used in the clinic required 3.5 minutes (totally manual record), whereas when the automated record could be consulted for laboratory results (X-ray and EKG results were still in the paper record), only 2 minutes were required.

Garrett et al. studied the impact of the Total Medical Record (TMR) system at Duke on the efficiency and quality of care in a renal clinic. When computer-generated medical record summaries and flowsheets were provided in place of the standard medical record, physicians spent less time reviewing charts before encounters, more time generating a computerized prescription, the same amount of time interacting with the patient, and achieved a 13 percent time savings overall. It should be noted that handwritten notes from the encounter form were transcribed into the system, though when the clerical time was included the person hours per visit were essentially unchanged (clerical time for transcription was approximately equal to the physician time savings). Physicians were less likely to overlook patient problems in computerized summaries and medication errors were also significantly reduced. (Since the study included no reminders or other prompting, the improvements were presumably due to the availability and format of prior data.)(31)

Several other studies offer further evidence of the impacts of computerized patient data on the process of care. In one controlled trial in a hospital emergency department, physician test ordering was compared with and without a printed flowsheet summary containing recent results for diagnostic studies generated by a computerized medical record system. When physicians had access to the flowsheet summary, they ordered fewer laboratory tests.(34)

Two studies of the Summary Time-Oriented Record (STOR) showed that the improved flow of information benefitted the clinical decision process.(30) In the first study, when a summary flowsheet from STOR was added to the standard medical record, physicians in an arthritis clinic were better able to predict the future symptoms and laboratory test results of their patients. When the paper medical record was no longer routinely pulled for a second study in a rheumatic diseases clinic, physicians were also better able to predict their patients' symptoms and test results. (They retained the option of obtaining the paper record, and did so for 26 percent of their patients, mostly for new patients, or for historical or test data not available in the computerized record.).

One study of a computerized record system in an outpatient geriatric practice followed patients over a period of a year to document impacts on the costs, quality, and outcomes of care.(35) Experimental patients had 25 percent more primary care visits, but fewer unscheduled visits. (No differences were observed in appointment utilization or costs of prescriptions and studies overall.) When hospitalizations were considered, the experimental group had significantly fewer hospital days and lower costs of hospital care. The authors estimated that the system resulted in a $596 per year savings in total costs per patient. They also found an increased ability to place patients with documented hypertension on therapy and better management of blood pressure.

(The evidence concerning the benefits of patient care information systems on ambulatory care comes mostly from studies of ambulatory medical record systems. Many of these take advantage of the patient database to provide rule-based prompting and reminders. Because of the difficulty of sorting out impacts due solely to improved information access from those attributable to decision support, the substantial benefits reported for these systems are discussed under *Contributions of System Decision Support*.)

Improved Information Access–Inpatient Care

Much of the research on the benefits of patient care information systems in inpatient settings has focused on nursing processes and the impacts on documentation and time devoted to information-related tasks. Interpreting this experience is complicated by the differences in baseline settings, systems, and approaches to implementation. Some of the evidence relates to the impacts of specialized nursing systems or more comprehensive systems used primarily to support the patient management tasks of nurses. As we evolve the concept of patient care information systems further, specialized support to nursing will be replaced by computer support to all staff involved in the care of inpatients. Many of the large-scale studies of early hospital information systems were also completed 12 to 20 years ago.(36-42) Therefore, care should be taken in extrapolating from most studies to specific settings today. Generally, however, the evidence does point to improvements in the many information-intensive tasks of caring for inpatients and is indicative of the direction of changes achievable in settings that lack advanced patient care information systems today.

One common finding in most studies is the improved quality and accuracy of nursing documentation. Once nursing assessment, care planning, and charting are supported, the structure of displays and worksheets and system prompts and edits all contribute to help reduce errors of omission in charting (such as not including reasons for nursing interventions not accomplished, site and reason for PRN medications administered). In one site with bedside access to a comprehensive system, nurses' charting of patient response to pain medication increased from 75.5 to 90 percent of the time and charting of findings from lung auscultation increased from 10 to 90 percent of the time.(43) Another study reported that date and time were included in documentation more reliably.(44)

Other impacts include increased quality and number of nursing observations, contributing to more complete documentation. One recent study involving the addition of automated nursing notes to a patient care information system revealed a slight time savings for creating computer-based notes, but a significant increase in the amount of data in the computerized assessment.(45) Another study of nurse charting in a general medical unit revealed that the charting and reevaluation of care plan actions increased from 19 to 38 percent to 55 to 66 percent following implementation of this application.(44)

Early hospital information systems were focused on order communication and charge capture for inpatient services. Consequently, results of the studies of these early systems reported increased charge capture and timeliness of order transmittal to ancillary departments such as the laboratory and pharmacy.(36) Increased timeliness of order receipt was also the rationale for decreased length of patient stay: If services could be initiated sooner, diagnostic results would be available sooner, necessary services coordinated, and treatments administered sooner. Decreases in length of stay were observed in several sites including El Camino Hospital where the issue was studied extensively in government-sponsored formal evaluations.(36,41,46)

Inpatient nursing is information-intensive, and manual procedures involve transcription and extensive record-keeping to manage nursing tasks and chart results and observations. Patient care information systems that capture physician orders and support the nursing process can eliminate redundant clerical tasks such as transcribing orders from the chart onto laboratory request slips and the patient Kardex. Several studies have explored changes in the amount of time nurses devote to information management and communication activities relative to time devoted to direct patient care.

Generally, the amount of time spent on indirect activities (nondirect care) is found to decline. In one study of changes due to computerized nurse charting, time devoted to paperwork decreased 9 percent.(44) In another study of the introduction of nurse charting and physical assessment, the amount of time spent on documentation increased from 27 to 36 percent, but time devoted to verbal communication decreased from 33 to 14 percent.(47) In the classic study years ago at El Camino, the portion of shift nurse time devoted to medications, communication, and reports/conferences declined. On average, nurse time devoted to clerical and communication activities for each patient/shift decreased from 22.7 minutes to 18.8 minutes.(42) A recent study of a care documentation system with bedside terminals revealed that time spent on nursing notes and care planning decreased from 60.6 minutes per patient per day before the system was installed to 33 minutes.(48)

Nursing time freed up from clerical and communication tasks is sometimes (37,47) but not always (38,39,44,48,49) devoted to direct patient care. These mixed findings convey several lessons. First, taking advantage of time savings requires a concerted effort to redesign work processes and reallocate tasks among members of the care team. The final results used in the economic analysis for El Camino(40) resulted from a work redesign program, and experience in other sites has confirmed that the desired redirection of time is not automatically a consequence of reduced paperwork.(38,48,50) Second, studies of nursing time are complicated and, because system implementation takes time, often involve taking measurements months or years apart to document the "before" and "after." This makes it difficult to control adequately for differences in medical and nursing practice, patient acuity, etc., in analyzing and interpreting results of these studies.(51,52)

Some studies have reported that labor savings can result in reduced overtime for nurses, which translates into direct cost savings for the hospital(53,54). In one study, 86 percent of overtime was required for nurses to complete documentation tasks.(50) Since patient care information systems have been shown to save time for this task, it is possible that the savings in overtime have accrued from this feature. However, systems can also save considerable time in collecting information concerning patient location, status, problems, incomplete activities, etc., to report to nursing staff for the next shift. In one study, each nurse spent nearly 42 minutes per shift preparing for report at the end of the shift.(50) Computer-generated summaries of up-to-date patient information can eliminate this labor-intensive step.(55) The studies at El Camino also revealed that the time for giving report declined by 20 to 82 percent on the six nursing units studied.(39)

Bedside terminals offer additional benefits over access at the central nursing station. The major benefit to the nursing process is the ability to chart vital signs and medications directly into the system at the bedside rather than handwriting the information and then "charting" it again at the nursing station. In addition, charting may occur closer to the time the nursing care was completed.(52) One study compared bedside with central system access (one terminal for each four patients) in an ICU. With bedside terminals, nurses reported spending less time waiting for terminals and were able to complete documentation within 30 minutes of the activity more often. Nurses felt bedside (direct) charting was more accurate, and over time bedside access increased the time for patient care.(56) Another study of the introduction of bedside access in three hospitals reported improvements in discharge teaching documentation and patient recall (14 percent), decreased patient use of nurse call systems, and reduced need for nurse overtime amounting to 26 minutes per nurse each shift.(57)

Relatively few studies have attempted to quantify the impacts of inpatient system support for physicians. At El Camino, physician time was measured in the baseline, but estimated by physicians after the system had been installed. Many (62 percent) of the physicians believed they were spending more time writing orders (performing order entry in the system), in chart review (68 percent), and in obtaining test results (43 percent).(42) Physician order entry has often been resisted because of the time required (58), and this undoubtedly influences the net impact for physicians when they are entering orders.

In our studies, physicians have reported spending less time searching for information when patient data are available on a computer (survey results are discussed in Chapter 3). In a study of the effect of the same patient care information system on information availability, physicians were 2.6 times more likely to have the information they needed for their patients when they arrived on the inpatient unit. When information was missing in the baseline (presystem), they reported spending time looking for information 39 percent of the time, ordering a repeat laboratory test or radiology examination 4.6 percent of the time, and delaying a decision about discharge 1.4 percent of the time.(10)

Systems that capture orders, results, and information about patient measurements (vital signs, fluid intake and output) can provide summaries (rounds reports) for physicians to use when they are rounding on inpatient units.(59-61) These are analogous to nursing change-of-shift reports in that they can compile and summarize up-to-date information that physicians need as they reassess patient status and consider changes in care strategy each day. No formal time studies are available to quantify how much physician time system compilations such as these can save, but they clearly save time and are likely to be more complete and accurate than handwritten notes compiled from patient charts and manual flowsheets and even from system terminals. (Rounds reports and other design features of patient care information systems that can add value to information access are discussed further in Chapter 4.)

Contributions of System Decision Support

Some of the greatest potential contributions of patient care information systems result from the combination of patient data with a knowledge base to produce patient-specific options or recommendations for diagnosis and treatment. Decision support is one area where patient care information systems can add enormous value over even the complete paper medical record or separate departmental systems. Computers can reliably correlate and interpret large volumes of patient data, applying rules to detect undesirable trends and events, and offering reminders and messages about diagnostic and therapeutic possibilities that may have been overlooked.(62) This contribution has led to an observation that patient care information systems are "informating" rather than merely automating the medical record because the databases provide an opportunity to enhance both the quality and efficiency of health care through increased analysis of care processes.(63) In the last 20 years, considerable evidence has emerged concerning the value of this support to patient management.(64,65)

Alerts

One type of decision support is geared to alerting physicians and nurses to potentially serious situations where delays in responding could be critical. One type of alert is dangerous conflicts in, or contraindications for interventions. The most common of these detect potential drug-allergy and drug-drug interactions. These alerts are available in stand-alone pharmacy systems, as well as many patient care information systems that capture medication orders. The database must contain medical orders for the patient and information on patient allergies, and the system reviews current orders using knowledge about possible interactions, and then provides displayed or printed messages to alert physicians, pharmacists and/or members of the care team when potential problems are detected. Another type of medication-related alert relies upon algorithms that combine factors such as patient age and weight to detect orders that contain potential dosing errors.

Another type of alert screens laboratory results for changes in patient status that may require a change in medication treatment or other intervention. Decision support in this case requires that laboratory test results be available in the data-base, and the system applies rules based on normal limits and preset alert limits to detect patient situations that should be reviewed. For example, the system may scan potassium levels obtained in the laboratory for patients receiving oral potassium, arterial and venous blood gas findings to detect hypoxemia, etc. The richer the patient database, the more opportunities exist for the system to detect potential problems.

The benefits of system-generated alerts were studied in one hospital with a patient care information system that had a rich clinical patient database and 86 types of drug-drug, drug-allergy, and drug-laboratory alerts for inpatients. The system offered both "action-oriented" and "informational" alerts (important, but not requiring an immediate response). During one 2-year period, the system generated alerts for 4 percent of the patients and 0.68 percent of drug orders; drug-laboratory alerts accounted for 55.5 percent, drug-drug orders for 36.3 percent, and drug-allergy for 8.2 percent of all alerts. Physicians complied with all of the "action-oriented" alerts. Based on a review of the experience with the 24 most beneficial alerts, clinical pharmacists reviewed cases in which the alert resulted in a change in patient care and estimated total benefits of $339,752 and a 4:1 benefit to cost ratio for the system.(66)

Another example of the benefits of alerts comes from a time-series controlled study of computer-generated alerts concerning renal function in hospitalized patients with nephrotoxic or renally excreted medications.(67) Researchers tracked instances in which rules concerning rising creatinine levels were met in patients on designated medications and the time between the availability of laboratory results and a change in the triggering medication or dose. During the study period, physicians involved in the patient's care were sent an alert message via electronic mail. Responses occurred on average 21.1 hours sooner when physicians received the computer-generated message.

Reminders and Recommendations

Patient care information systems can also provide feedback about care processes, remembering tasks that should be accomplished or suggesting a diagnosis or treatment protocol that may apply to a particular patient. Like the alerts discussed earlier, this type of decision support requires consistent capture of the necessary patient information and rules that describe the condition (one or a combination of patient-specific facts) and frame the reminder message. Computer feedback to the physician can either be via printed reports or on-line during user interaction with the system.

Most computerized reminder rules are triggered when the system detects that a patient meets the condition(s) defined in the rule (i.e., has an appointment today and is on a particular medication that should be reviewed, is overdue for a particular health screening procedure, has a diagnostic finding that requires follow-up, or has documented health risk factors that match a protocol for further testing). A number of studies have documented that physicians do respond when they are reminded that patients meet such conditions.

Computerized reminders can increase the success rate in following up on abnormal diagnostic results. An early study of reminders in the COSTAR system showed that follow-up of positive throat cultures within 10 days increased from 90 to 100 percent.(68) Another reminder in COSTAR resulted in improved follow-up of patients with newly discovered elevated blood pressure. When the system noted the absence of two additional blood pressure readings for a patient in the 6 months following the recording of the initial high reading, a system-generated reminder was sent to the patient's physician. Physicians who received these reminders attempted or achieved follow-up 84 percent of the time versus 25 percent of the time for control patients.(69)

Preventive medicine provides a good example of some of the information management challenges of incorporating clinical guidelines into medical practice and the improvements that can be achieved with computer-generated reminders. Matching patients with the appropriate preventive procedures requires two different types of information:

• The guidelines typically vary according to the age and sex of the patient at a minimum and often additional demographic characteristics (such as race), family history (e.g., family history of breast cancer), and/or comorbidity

(e.g., diabetes) so that identifying/remembering the appropriate guideline for each case can be difficult.(70)
- Preventive medicine/primary care guidelines call for periodic services at recommended time intervals (e.g., each year, every 3 years). In order to determine whether recommended services are due (or overdue), a physician/provider also needs access to complete information about the dates of the most recent relevant preventive services.

Once the necessary patient information is available in the database of a patient care information system, rules can be created to scan patient data for compliance with a potentially unlimited number of guidelines for care and to provide appropriate reminders. Computer-generated reminders can take the form of physician reminders (printed or on-line) and patient reminders or mailers. In one study, results for physician reminders, patient reminders, and both types of reminders combined were compared for five recommended preventive services. Adherence to guidelines increased for each type of reminder. The largest increases were observed when the two forms of reminders were used together and included an increase in fecal occult blood testing from 9.3 to 38.1 percent and an increase in compliance with guidelines for mammography from 11.4 to 27.1 percent.(71)

Impressive results have also been obtained for improving influenza vaccination performance with computer-generated reminders.(72,73) In one 3-year trial of preventive care reminders, physicians who received reminders vaccinated eligible patients twice as often as control physicians. Researchers also tracked emergency room visits requiring chest X-ray studies, blood gas determinations, and hospitalizations in vaccinated versus unvaccinated patients and concluded that vaccination reduced morbidity during the subsequent influenza season by 10 to 30 percent.(74)

Some experience has also been gained in implementing numerous system reminders simultaneously within a medical practice. In one randomized trial, a computer record system containing 1,490 care rules was used to generate reports with appropriate reminder messages for patients with appointments in an internal medicine clinic. Reminder sheets were given to physicians on study teams, and the system kept records of the indications for actions for both study and control patients. During the course of the 2-year study, the computer found indications for at least one clinical action in more than 90 percent of all scheduled patient encounters. Residents who received reminders responded to clinical indications in their patients 49 percent of the time versus 29 percent of the time for residents who did not receive reminders. Residents in study groups were two to four times more likely to apply preventive care to their eligible patients. The computer reminders had no discernible effects on the patient outcomes examined.(75)

Several studies have followed patients in a particular clinic setting with computerized records over a period of time to detect changes in processes and outcomes. One of these compared care of patients in a cardiac, pulmonary, and renal clinic with and without a summary produced by an automated medical record system including prompts relating to good practice to supplement the traditional record during patient encounters. Over the 2-year period, experimental patients underwent more laboratory procedures and/or were given (or had reviewed) more diets. Of eight procedures recommended in three disease areas, four were performed more frequently in experimental than in control patients. Some improvements in patient outcomes were also observed.(32)

Another study compared the use of an electronic medical record and special forms and checklists designed to aid in the care of patients with HIV infection with and without system-generated alerts and reminders that call attention to clinical events and aid in carrying out responses such as ordering a test or prescribing a particular medication. Physicians in the intervention group were able to comply with clinical guidelines more than twice as rapidly and completely than physicians who did not receive the decision support. In addition to more primary care interventions, the support was also associated with more complete documentation and more ambulatory care encounters, but no difference in the overall costs of care.(76)

At Latter Day Saints (LDS) Hospital, decision support is focused on inpatient care and includes the ability to embed protocols for patient care that are triggered by events recorded in the patient database. One application is ventilator management protocols for patients with adult respiratory distress syndrome. Based on patient data captured by the system, instructions were automatically generated and available on bedside terminals in the ICU. Providing system-generated instructions in this way increased compliance with the protocol and patient survival rate.(77,78)

In another application for management of patients with deep vein thrombosis, the physician interacts directly with the system, entering the clinical problem to be addressed, and the system prepares a suggested patient-specific treatment plan based on knowledge-based guidelines and patient information. Initial studies indicate that a higher proportion of system suggestions are appropriate than management decisions made by attending physicians.(79)

Support to Research and Development of Improved Practices

Comprehensive patient databases that include information on patient characteristics and health history for large numbers of patients provide a reservoir that can be tapped for important purposes other than direct care. Much of the information needed for research and quality management is the same as needed for patient care. If the data are stored so that they can be queried, aggregated, and downloaded, and tools are provided for extracting and analyzing information about subgroups of patients or health care episodes based upon common attributes, patient care information systems can make substantial contributions to research and examination of care delivery to develop better practices.

Depending upon the scope of patient data available, enhanced access to patient data can benefit categories of research ranging from clinical research to quality of care evaluation, examination of patterns or variations in care, and studies of utilization and outcomes.(80)

The ease and speed of obtaining information is one obvious advantage. One example in the literature describes a small research study focused on the association between homelessness and admission to an inpatient alcohol treatment program.(81) The author reported that obtaining the results from an automated medical record system took only 5 minutes, whereas obtaining the information from traditional records "would literally take months."

Accuracy and completeness are also improved. The traditional method for assembling patient information needed for research is to extract information from patient medical records, record it on specially designed forms, and enter the data obtained into a computer for analysis. (This approach is obviously time-consuming and costly.) In one study of data abstracted from records for a clinical trial, manually recorded data contained at least one error of transcription in 17 percent of cases (versus none for computer-generated data) and was incomplete in 35 percent of the cases examined (versus 2 percent for computerized data).(82)

Researchers in one major teaching hospital with a robust clinical database have provided impressive evidence of the benefits derived from their ability to examine processes and outcomes:

- A hospital computer system that included alerts designed to detect and respond to adverse drug events also created a database concerning the alerts generated. This information was used to refine the rules for notifying physicians, with the result that the incidence of adverse drug events was decreased further.(83)
- Information on hospital-acquired infections from a hospital clinical system was used to identify risk factors for infection, develop a model for infection prediction, and acquire knowledge concerning likely pathogens and appropriate antibiotics. This permitted incorporating knowledge-based rules in the system to identify at-risk patients and assist in the selection of appropriate antibiotics.(84)
- Using information captured in a clinical database, researchers studied the impact of the timing of prophylactic antibiotics on the risk of infection in surgery patients, and were able to establish that administration 2 hours before surgery reduced the risk of wound infection.(85)

In many hospitals that lack advanced patient care information systems, the most comprehensive database available is the hospital discharge database, which contains data assembled about each admission primarily for obtaining reimbursement. Similar data are routinely collected in a standardized format to include on bills for ambulatory services and are captured in the databases of billing systems. These data are already collected and available in electronic form, and they include coded information about patient diagnoses and procedures. In the absence of other consistently collected electronic information about hospital stays or ambulatory encounters, these billing databases are the best available data source for studying the quality of care and clinical outcomes.

Several studies have addressed problems with the reliability and validity of insurance claims data as the source of patient care documentation:

- Researchers in a tertiary care hospital studied the concordance of information concerning patients with ischemic heart disease in two databases: insurance claims data and data in a clinical database. In more than half of the cases examined, claims data did not include prognostically important conditions (such as diabetes mellitus) that relate to underlying illness or severity.(86)
- When discharge abstracts were compared with medical records in five hospitals, 82 percent of the records differed from the abstract in at least one item and 22 percent of items in abstracts were in error. Correction of errors in abstracts was projected to change diagnosis-related group assignment in 19 percent of the cases examined.(87)
- In a family practice affiliated with a medical school, progress notes were reviewed by physicians to extract information concerning level of service, diagnosis, and procedures, and the results were compared with the corresponding information contained in the billing database. Agreement between billing data and progress notes on level of service and the number of diagnoses was poor. Billing forms listed only 69 percent of diagnoses, and had diagnoses corresponding to those from the encounter note only 60 percent of the time.(88)

These results underscore the importance of evolving patient care information systems to the point that they provide the patient information needed for research on patterns and outcomes of care.

Physicians as Direct System Users

As clinical support has evolved in the direction of the ultimate patient care information system, physicians have become more involved as direct users. From terminals in patient care areas, they can query systems directly to obtain the information they need, and in some cases physicians also enter orders and documentation into systems. The Institute of Medicine study(9) and others(89, 90) have called for integrating patient care information systems into the basic processes of care and patient management in order to gain the maximum benefits. If physicians and other providers enter orders and care plans themselves, this streamlines the process, eliminates the need for transcription and attendant errors and delays, and leverages the full value of decision support. This section reviews the rationale for involving physicians in using patient care information systems interactively and the current evidence of the benefits to be gained.

Physicians initiate or approve most health care services. Assuming that they control all surgical procedures, hospitalizations, and prescription drugs, they control 90 percent of health care expenditures.(91) Therefore, to the extent that better access to patient data and patient management tools offer improvements in how and when health care resources are utilized, these must be available at the point of production to achieve true efficiencies and quality.(92)

By consulting systems directly, physicians can have the benefit of the most up-to-date information concerning their patients. The sentinel automated medical record systems have provided printed summaries for patient encounters as the primary source of patient data and reminders.(25,30,31,93) Summaries printed the night before the encounter reflect all available information, and the reminders generated do influence physician behavior, as discussed previously in this chapter. However, when physicians do not interact with the system during the visit, decision support can only be driven by history rather than address any new information obtained during the encounter; this suggests that additional benefits can be gained when decision support is supplied interactively.(35)

Before decision support can address patient management decisions concurrently as the physician is making them, orders need to be captured in real time. Some improvements can be gained when the decision support message is received by staff such as pharmacists.(94) Periodic feedback to physicians concerning their ordering practices has also been shown to influence practice, as evidenced in one study concerning the prescribing of generic drugs.(95) However, these indirect mechanisms become unwieldy and costly as the scope of decision support expands, and are not likely to be practical or effective for large numbers of interventions. Furthermore, one study that compared the effectiveness of delayed feedback versus immediate reminders concerning 13 preventive care protocols revealed that compliance increased at double the rate for some of the protocols, and by half again as much for others, when physicians had the feedback available during the encounter.(96)

Impressive results have been obtained when physician order entry is combined with decision support. In one study, physicians entered orders for all outpatient diagnostic tests into a patient care information system; the physicians who received displays of charges for each item and total charges for the patient ordered 14 percent fewer tests, resulting in total charges per patient that were 13 percent lower than those of their colleagues who received no information on charges.(97)

Another study from the same academic medical center involved interns ordering inpatient tests and medications from special menus designed to encourage cost-effective ordering: charges were displayed for each item, the most cost-effective tests were displayed for the specific patient's problem, and reasonable testing intervals were indicated (e.g., three times a week rather than daily). Inpatient charges were lower (12.7 percent) and lengths of stay shorter (10.5 percent) for patients whose orders were managed using the order entry menus containing this information.(98)

In another study with the same patient care information system, statistical equations were used to predict which patients would have abnormal results on eight commonly ordered laboratory tests. Physicians who received prompts concerning the predictions ordered 8.8 percent fewer tests for their patients, with the result that testing patterns were shifted to higher-risk patients.(99)

When real-time entry of outpatient prescriptions is also linked electronically to the pharmacies where patients obtain their medications, a further benefit is information about patient compliance. This was an unanticipated benefit of physician order entry into the Department of Defense Composite Health Care System. At one of the initial hospital sites, physicians entered orders for prescriptions into the system that were transmitted to the pharmacy for dispensing. When patients failed to pick up prescriptions within 5 days, noncompliance was noted in the system. Of the 1,100 to 1,500 prescriptions processed each day, 1.84 percent were unclaimed. Information concerning noncompliant patients could be obtained from the system, and system data permitted examining noncompliance for different categories of medications and different clinics.(100)

Clearly, as more decision aids and patient management tools are incorporated into patient care information systems, the incentives for involving physicians as direct users will increase. Much of the physician resistance to becoming active system users can be attributed to the increased time required to accomplish tasks such as entering orders and patient notes. The accumulating evidence concerning the benefits to be gained underscores the importance of resolving these design issues to minimize user time and maximize the value of patient care information systems in patient management. (Chapter 4 reviews some of the design prerequisites that can lead to more acceptable systems.)

Where Benefits Assessment Goes from Here

Assessment Research

When early patient care information systems were being developed and installed, there was a flurry of research on the impacts of these innovations on care processes and costs, much of it sponsored by the government. Since that time, much of the interest in the benefits of systems that support patient care has been focused on identifying sufficient benefits to justify the investment, either within the health care organization or to external review bodies.

Now, the landscape has changed significantly. The new incentives of managed care make the real value of investments in patient care information systems their ability to enable positive health care outcomes for the health care enterprise. The ability to manage patient care is dependent upon the quality of information access and information management tools. Hence, the questions involving investments in patient care information systems have shifted from "whether" and "when" to "what" and "how."

Benefits assessment is more important than ever to demonstrate successful models of matching the technology of the patient care information system with the dynamics and business of the health care organization. Benefits studies can provide the evidence needed to gauge reasonable expectations of improvements achievable in different settings and with different approaches to system design and implementation.

Much of the published research on advanced patient care information systems comes from academic medical centers with programs in medical informatics. The systems in these centers are for the most part self-developed. The local interest in system design and a research orientation make these centers important contributors to advancing the state of the art of patient care information systems. Through published research the medical informatics community also plays a major role in sharing the lessons and successes of their efforts.

More research is needed, however, on the transferability of the successful systems in these sites to the community hospital and physician office practice environment. Differences in staffing, operation, and system expertise may require other models for physician interaction, tailoring of decision support functions to accommodate local best practices, embedding decision support into clinical practice, and capturing patient information most efficiently. Research is needed to address topics such as these in the other health care settings that will be part of the integrated care delivery systems of the future to expand the knowledge base about successful strategies for implementing patient care information systems and the impacts on processes and outcomes of care.

Published research is only useful as a guide for others if the publications include sufficient detail about the objectives and constraints of the patient care information system project, the routine operations of patient care before and after introduction of the computer, the specific system applications and involvement of different care givers as direct users, the problems encountered, and the lessons learned.(101) If researchers describe more of these topics in detail, readers will be better able to understand the relevance to their systems projects and health care settings.

Benefits Assessment as a System Report Card

Within each health care organization, formal assessment of benefits can play an important role in ensuring that objectives for the patient care information system are achieved. Focused on indicators for processes that are key to the success of the health care enterprise, benefits assessment can provide the measurements used to track progress and to identify opportunities for improvement. Assessment results at formal checkpoints can be combined with constantly taking the pulse of users, their evolving needs and their suggestions of enhancements and improvements to target parts of the business where fine tuning or rethinking of business processes and/or system support can further improve performance. When used in this way in combination with change management, benefits assessment can provide a useful report card on the extent to which the potential of a patient care information system is being realized and a structured approach for continually improving the value of the system to care delivery.(102)

References

1. Woolhandler S, Himmelstein DU, Lewontin JP. Administrative costs in U.S. hospitals. The New England Journal of Medicine 1993;329:400-403.
2. Holbrook J. A computerized audit of 15,009 emergency department records. Annals of Emergency Medicine 1990;19:139-144.
3. Tufo HM, Speidel JJ. Problems with medical records. Medical Care 1971;IX:509-517.
4. Romm FJ, Putnam SM. The validity of the medical record. Medical Care 1981;19:310-315.
5. Safran C, Rury C, Rind DM, Taylor WC. A computer-based outpatient medical record for a teaching hospital. M.D. Computing 1991; 8(5):291-299.
6. Arthur D. Little, Inc. Evaluation of a Hospital Information System in Military Medical Treatment Facilities. Volumes I-VII. Report to the TRIMIS Program Office, Bethesda, MD, 1983.
7. Pories WJ. Is the medical record dangerous to our health? North Carolina Medical Journal 1990;51:47-55.
8. Kuperman GJ, Maack BB, Bauer K, et al. Innovations and research review: The impact of the HELP computer system on the LDS Hospital paper medical record. Topics in Health Record Management 1991;12:76-85.
9. Campbell JR, Seelig CB, Wigton RS, et al. Clinic function and computerized ambulatory records: a concurrent study with conventional records. Proceedings of the 12th Annual SCAMC. IEEE Publishers, 1988;745-748.
10. CHCS Program Office. Interim Benefits Assessment of the Composite Health Care System. Arthur D. Little, Inc., Report under Contract MDA 903-88-C-0064. Falls Church VA: CHCS Program Office, 1992.
11. Selker HP, Beshansky JR, Paulker SG, et al. The epidemiology of delays in a teaching hospital. The development and use of a tool that detects unnecessary hospital days. Medical Care 1989;27:112-129.
12. Palmer, RH, Strain R, Rothrock JK, et al. Evaluation of operational failures in clinical decision making. Medical Decision Making 1983;3:299-310.
13. Banks NJ, Palmer RH, Berwick DM. Improving the quality of ambulatory health care with enhanced medical information systems: Using the computer to diagnose faulty clinical processes. Journal of Medical Systems 1990;14:345-349.
14. Harvard Medical Practice Study. Patients, Doctors, and Lawyers: Medical Injury, Malpractice Litigation, and Patient Compensation in New York. Cambridge, MA:Harvard Medical Practice Study, 1990.

15. Tate, KE. Gardner RM. Computers, quality, and the clinical laboratory: a look at critical value reporting. Proceedings of the 17th Annual SCAMC. McGraw-Hill, Inc., 1994;193-197.
16. Melmon KL. Preventable drug reactions - Causes and cures. New England Journal of Medicine 1971;284:1361-1368.
17. Bates DW, Leape L, Petrycki S. Drug-related adverse events in hospitalized adults. Clinical Research 1991;596A.
18. Zielstorff RD, McHugh ML, Clinton J. Computer Design Criteria for Systems That Support the Nursing Process. Kansas City MO: American Nurses' Association, 1988.
19. Dick RD, Steen EB [eds.] The Computer-Based Patient Record. An Essential Technology for Health Care. Washington, DC: National Academy Press, 1991.
20. Jydstrup RA, Gross MJ. Cost of information handling in hospitals. Health Services Research 1966;Winter:235-271.
21. Fries, JF. Alternatives in medical record formats. Medical Care 1974; XII:871-881.
22. Clayton PD and Nobel, JJ. Costs and Cost Justification for Integrated Information Systems in Medicine. Proceedings for the IMIA Working Conference on Hospital Information Systems: Scope and Design Architecture. September 9-11, 1991, Goettingen, Germany; Bakken Ehlers Bryant and Hammond Editors.
23. Overhage JM, Tierney WM, McDonald CJ, et al. How do interns spend their days: a time-motion study of internal medicine interns. Clinical Research 1991;39:794A.
24. Lurie N, Rank B, Parenti C, et al. How do house officers spend their nights? A time study of internal medicine house staff on call. New England Journal of Medicine 1989;25:1673-1677.
25. McDonald CJ, Murray R, Jeris D, et al. A computer-based record and clinical monitoring system for ambulatory care. American Journal of Public Health 1977;67:240-245.
26. Mamlin JJ, Baker DH. Combined time-motion and work sampling study in a general medicine clinic. Medical Care 1973;11:449-456.
27. Arthur D. Little, Inc. Preliminary Economic Analysis of Equipment Enhancements to the Tri-Service Radiology System at Naval Hospital, Bethesda. Report to the TRIMIS Program Office, February 1984.
28. Zielstorff RD, Roglieri JL, Marble KD, et al. Experience with a computer-based medical record for nurse practitioners in ambulatory care. Computers and Biomedical Research 1977;10:61-74.
29. Campbell JR, Givner N, Seelig CB, et al. Computerized medical records and clinic functions. M.D. Computing 1989;6:282-287.
30. Whiting-O'Keefe QE, Simborg DW, Epstein WV, et al. A computerized summary can provide more information than the standard medical record. Journal of the American Medical Association 1985;254:1185-1192.

31. Garrett LE, Hammond WE, Stead WW. The effects of computerized medical records on provider efficiency and quality of care. Methods of Information in Medicine 1986;25:151-157.
32. Rogers JL, Haring OM, Wortman PL, et al. Medical information systems: Assessing impact in the areas of hypertension, obesity, and renal disease. Medical Care 1982;20:63-74.
33. Barnett GO. The application of computer-based medical-record systems in ambulatory practice. New England Journal of Medicine 1984;310:1643-1650.
34. Wilson GA, McDonald CJ, McCabe GP. The effect of immediate access to a computerized medical record on physician test ordering: a controlled clinical trial in the emergency room. American Journal of Public Health 1982;72:698-702.
35. Hammond KW, Prather RJ, Date VV, et al. A provider-interactive medical record system can favorably influence costs and quality of care. Computers in Biology and Medicine 1990;20:267-279.
36. Schmitz HH. An evaluation of a modular hospital information system. Hospital Progress 1972;53:70-76.
37. Simborg DW, MacDonald LK, Liebman JS, et al. Ward information-management system: an evaluation. Computers and Biomedical Research 1972;5:484-497.
38. Tolbert SH, Pertuz AE. Study shows how computerization affects nursing activities in ICU. Hospitals 1977;51:79-84.
39. Barrett JF, Barnum RA, Gordon BB, et al. Evaluation of the Implementation of a Medical Information System in a General Community Hospital. Battelle Columbus Laboratories Report to the Bureau of Health Services Research. Springfield, VA: National Technical Information Service 1975;Report PB 248-340.
40. Gall JE, Cook M, Greming J, et al. Demonstration and Evaluation of a Total Hospital Information System. Report to the National Center for Health Services Research. Springfield, VA: National Technical Information Service 1975; Report PB 262 106.
41. Barrett JP, Hersch PL, Caswell RJ. Evaluation of the Implementation of the Technicon Medical Information System at El Camino Hospital. Part II. Economic Trend Analysis. Columbus, OH: Battelle, 1979.
42. Battelle Memorial Institute. Evaluation of the Implementation of a Medical Information System in a General Community Hospital. Vol. II. Evaluation Studies and Analyses. Report to Bureau of Health Services Research. Springfield, VA:National Technical Information Service 1973;Report PB-232 785.
43. Martin GT, Baker G. Measuring the benefits of bedside systems. Healthcare Informatics 1993;May:26-30.
44. Johnson DS, Burkes M, Sitting D, et al. Evaluation of the effects of computerized nurse charting. Proceedings of the 11th Annual SCAMC, IEEE Publishers, 1987;363-367.

45. Grewal R, Arcus J, Bowen J, et al. Design and development of an automated nursing note. MEDINFO 92, Amsterdam:Elsevier (North-Holland) 1992;1054-1058.
46. Kwon IW, Vogler, TK, Adam J, et al. Cost effective analysis of the use of a computer in health care. Computers in Hospitals 1980;Nov/Dec:22-23.
47. Hinson DK, Huether SW, Blaufuss JA, et al. Measuring the impact of a clinical nursing information system on one nursing unit. Proceedings of the 17th Annual SCAMC. McGraw-Hill, Inc., 1994;203-210.
48. Balcerak KJ, Lambert AA. The effect of computerized documentation systems on selected nursing activities. Proceedings of the 1994 Annual HIMSS Conference. Chicago, IL: Healthcare Information and Management Systems Society, 1994;4:295-309.
49. Schmitz HH, Ellerbrake RP, Williams TM. Study evaluates effects of new communication system. Hospitals 1976;50:129-134.
50. Kahl K, Ivancil L, Fuhrmann M, et al. Measuring the savings achieved by use of bedside terminals. Proceedings of the 1991 Annual HIMSS Conference. Chicago, IL: American Hospital Association, 1991;145-161.
51. Staggers N. Using computers in nursing. Documented benefits and needed studies. Computers in Nursing 1988;6(4):164-169.
52. Hendrickson G, Kovner CT. Effects of computers on nursing resource use. Computers in Nursing 1990;8(1):16-22.
53. Pesce J. Bedside terminals: MEDTAKE. M.D. Computing 1988;5:16-21.
54. Lower MS, Nauert LB. Charting: the impact of bedside computers. Nursing Management 1992;23(7):40-44.
55. Hujcs M. Utilizing computer integration to assist nursing. Proceedings of the 14th Annual SCAMC. IEEE Publishers, 1990;894-897.
56. Halford G, Burkes M, Pryor TA. Measuring the impact of bedside terminals. Nursing Management 1989;20(7):41-45.
57. Cerne F. Information management study finds bedside terminals prove their worth. Hospitals 1989;63:72.
58. Massaro TA. Introducing physician order entry at a major academic medical center. II. Impact on medical education. Academic Medicine 1993;68:25-30.
59. McDonald CJ, Tierney WM, Overhage JM, et al. The Regenstreif Medical Record System: 20 years of experience in hospitals, clinics, and neighborhood health centers. MD Computing 1992:9:206-217.
60. Michael PA. Physician-directed software design: the role of utilization statistics and user input in enhancing HELP results review capabilities. Proceedings of the 17th Annual SCAMC. McGraw-Hill, Inc.,1994;107-111.
61. Bradshaw KE, Gardner RM, Clemmer TP, et al. Physician decision-making - Evaluation of data used in a computerized ICU. International Journal of Clinical Monitoring and Computing 1984:1:81-94.
62. Johnson DS, Ranzenberger, Herbert RD. A computerized alert program for acutely ill patients. Journal of Nursing Administration, 1980;June 26-35.

63. Friedman BA. Informating not automating the medical record. Journal of Medical Systems 1989;13:221-225.
64. Haynes BH, Walker CJ. Computer-aided quality assurance. Archives of Internal Medicine 1987;147:1297-1303.
65. Langton KB, Johnston ME, Haynes RB, et al. A critical appraisal of the literature on the effects of computer-based clinical decision support systems on clinician performance and patient outcomes. Proceedings of the 16th Annual SCAMC. McGraw-Hill, Inc., 1993;626-630.
66. Gardner RM, Hulse RK, Larsen KG. Assessing the effectiveness of a computerized pharmacy system. Proceedings of the 14th Annual SCAMC. McGraw-Hill, Inc., 1990;668-672.
67. Rind DM, Safran C, Phillips RS, et al. The effect of computer-based reminders on the management of hospitalized patients with worsening renal function. Proceedings of the 15th Annual SCAMC. McGraw-Hill, Inc., 19;28-32.
68. Barnett GO. Winickoff R, Dorsey JL, et al. Quality assurance through automated monitoring and concurrent feedback using a computer-based medical information system. Medical Care 1978;16:962-973.
69. Barnett GO, Winickoff RN, Morgan MM, et al. A computer-based monitoring system for follow-up of elevated blood pressure. Medical Care 1983;21:400-408.
70. U.S. Preventive Services Task Force. Guide to Clinical Preventive Services. An Assessment of the Effectiveness of 169 Interventions, Baltimore, MD: Williams & Wilkins, 1989.
71. Ornstein SM, Garr DR, Jenkins RG, et al. Computer-generated physician and patient reminders. Tools to improve population adherence to selected preventive services. The Journal of Family Practice 1991;32:82-90.
72. Hutchison BG. Effect of computer-generated nurse/physician reminders on influenza immunization among seniors. Family Medicine 1989;21:433-437.
73. Barton MB, Schoenbaum SC. Improving influenza vaccination performance in an HMO setting: the use of computer-generated reminders and peer comparison feedback. American Journal of Public Health 1990;80:534-536.
74. McDonald CJ, Hui SL, Tierney WM. Effects of computer reminders for influenza vaccination on morbidity during influenza epidemics. M.D. Computing 1992;9:304-312.
75. McDonald CJ, Hui SL, Smith DM, et al. Reminders to physicians from an introspective computer medical record. Annals of Internal Medicine 1984;100:130-138.
76. Safran C, Rind DM, Davis RM, et al. An electronic medical record that helps care for patients with HIV infection. Proceedings of the 17th Annual SCAMC. McGraw-Hill, Inc., 1994;224-228.
77. Henderson S, East TD, Morris AH, et al. Performance evaluation of computerized clinical protocols for management of arterial hypoxemia in

ARDS patients. Proceedings of the 13th Annual SCAMC. IEEE Publishers, 1989;588-592.

78. Henderson S, Crapo RO, East TD, et al. Computerized clinical protocols in an intensive care unit: How well are they followed? Proceedings of the 14th Annual SCAMC. IEEE Publishers, 1990;284-288.

79. Lam SH. Implementation and evaluation of practice guidelines. Proceedings of the 17th Annual SCAMC. McGraw-Hill, Inc., 1994;253-257.

80. Davies AR. Health care researchers' Needs for computer-based patient records. In Ball MJ, Collen MF (eds) Aspects of the Computer-Based Patient Record. New York: Springer Verlag, 1992;46-56.

81. Chang MM. Clinician-entered computerized psychiatric triage records. Hospital and Community Psychiatry 1987;38:652-656.

82. Elting LS, Bodey GP. Evaluation of benefits derived from a computerized data management system for clinical trials data. Proceedings of the 15th Annual SCAMC. McGraw-Hill, Inc., 1992;48-52.

83. Evans RS, Pestonik SL, Classen DC, et al. Prevention of adverse drug events through computerized surveillance. Proceedings of the 16th Annual SCAMC. McGraw-Hill, Inc., 1993;437-441.

84. Evans RS, Burke JP, Pestonik SL, et al. Prediction of hospital infections and selection of antibiotics using an automated hospital database. Proceedings of the 14th Annual SCAMC. McGraw-Hill, Inc., 1990;663-667.

85. Classen DC, Evans RS, Pestonik SL, et al. The timing of prophylactic administration of antibiotics and the risk of surgical-wound infection. New England Journal of Medicine 1992; 326:281-286.

86. Jollis, JG, Ancukiewicz M, DeLong ER, et al. Discordance of databases designed for claims payment versus clinical information systems. Annals of Internal Medicine 1993;119:844-850.

87. Lloyd SS, Rissing R. Physician and coding errors in patient records. Journal of the American Medical Association 1985;254:1330-1336.

88. Horner RD, Paris JA, Purvis JR, et al. Accuracy of patient encounter and billing information in ambulatory care. The Journal of Family Practice 1991;33:593-598.

89. Government Accounting Office. Medical ADP Systems. Automated Records Hold Promise to Improve Patient Care. GAO/IMTEC-91-5. Washington, DC, 1991.

90. Work Group on Computerization of Patient Records. Toward a National Health Information Infrastructure. Report to the Secretary of the U.S. Department of Health and Human Services, April 1993.

91. Wilensky GR, Rossiter LF. The relative importance of physician-induced demand in the demand for medical care. Milbank Memorial Fund Quarterly 1983;61:252-277.

92. Nobel JJ. The health care professional's work station. International Journal of Bio-Medical Computing 1994;34(1-4):21-28.

93. Barnett GO. Computer-Stored Ambulatory Record. National Center for Health Services Research. NCHSR Research Digest Series, DHEW Publication No. (HRA) 76-3145, 1976.

94. Goldberg, DE. Baardsgaard G, Johnson MT, et al. Computer-based program for identifying medication orders requiring dosage modification based on renal function. American Journal of Hospital Pharmacy 1991;48:1965-1969.

95. Gehlbach SH, Wilkinson WE, Clapp NE. Improving drug prescribing in a primary care practice. Medical Care 1984;22:193-201.

96. Tierney WM, Hui SL, McDonald CJ. Delayed feedback of physician performance versus immediate reminders to perform preventive care. Medical Care 1986;24:659-666.

97. Tierney WM, Miller ME, McDonald CJ. The effect on test ordering of informing physicians of the charges for outpatient diagnostic tests. New England Journal of Medicine 1990;322:1499-1504.

98. Tierney WM, Miller ME, Overhage JM, et al. Physician inpatient order writing on microcomputer workstations. Journal of the American Medical Association 1993;269:379-383.

99. Tierney WM. McDonald CJ, Hui SL, et al. Computer predictions of abnormal test results. Effects on outpatient testing. Journal of the American Medical Association 1988;259:1194-1198.

100. Craghead RM, Wartski DM. An evaluation study of unclaimed prescriptions. Hospital Pharmacy 1991;26:616-632.

101. Zielstorff RD, Abraham IL, Werley HL, et al. Guidelines for reporting innovations in computer-based information systems for nursing. Computers in Nursing 1989;7(5):203-208.

102. Drazen EL. Beyond cost benefit: an assessment approach for the '90s. Proceedings of the 15th Annual SCAMC. McGraw-Hill, Inc., 1992;13-17.

2
Physicians' and Nurses' Acceptance of Computers

Erica L. Drazen

In the previous chapter, we outlined some of the potential benefits to be gained by using computers to support patient care. However, in order to influence the costs and outcomes of care by using computers, these systems must be accepted by physicians, nurses, and others who take care of patients.

Many studies have been conducted of physicians' and nurses' acceptance of computers, and even more folklore has circulated about whether and why these groups will welcome computer support for patient care delivery. In this chapter we will review this experience in order to identify key findings that may be useful in predicting future acceptance of computers.

There are three common measures of computer acceptance: user attitudes, actual use, and user satisfaction. User attitudes (assessed mainly among groups that have not used computers) was the most common measure in early studies. This measure was relevant when trying to predict whether computers would diffuse naturally into the health care environment or whether special efforts would be required to promote their use.

Once computers had been introduced into health care delivery, the most relevant question became, "Are these systems useful?" The two most common measures of usefulness were voluntary use of the computer instead of manual methods and user satisfaction. In situations where use of the system is mandatory, satisfaction is the only way to determine acceptance.

The largest body of reported information is related to attitudes toward computers. However, most of the research in this area is more than 5 years old. Since attitudes toward computers have no doubt changed, the findings of these studies may no longer be applicable. Moreover, since computers are being used successfully in many settings, the question of whether or not physicians and nurses will accept computers is probably no longer germane. We have included a synopsis of several of the early studies on attitudes toward computers for completeness, as well as to demonstrate that the common folklore about physician resistance to computers was not supported by study results. To reflect the evolution of attitudes, studies are presented in rough chronological sequence.

Attitudes Toward Computers

One of the earliest studies of physicians' attitudes toward computers was obtained in a 1980s survey of the views of Baltimore-area physicians, certified public accountants, lawyers, and pharmacists.(1) A survey was mailed to 500 people from each group (except CPAs because there were fewer than 500 in the area). A database of 521 total responses was examined to analyze the respondents' views on the benefits of computers, feelings about the depersonalizing effects of computers, and enthusiasm for using computers. All groups felt that some aspects of computers were positive (providing tools) and that other aspects were negative (depersonalization and difficulty in learning a computer language). CPAs and pharmacists were the most positive about computers, physicians were neutral, and lawyers were the most negative. Respondents who had used computers had more positive attitudes than those with no computer experience.

It is likely that in the early 1980s most physicians were unaware of the potential benefits of computers in clinical practice. In later studies, physicians reported more experience with computers, and physician attitudes documented in later studies were positive rather than neutral.(2-4) The overall feeling that the computer is a potentially useful tool was evident in this early research and was consistently documented in later studies.

In the early 1980s, an attitude survey was conducted of 85 physicians who had registered for a short tutorial in medical computing and informatics as well as a sample of 61 other academic and community-based physicians who were affiliated with a major teaching hospital.(2) More than 80 percent of the survey respondents indicated that they would accept computer systems to support medical records, hospital information systems, patient monitoring, diagnostic consults, and therapy consults. Only 32 percent thought computers were acceptable as a substitute for physicians. Physicians in medical specialties had higher acceptance ratings than surgeons. There were no differences in attitudes based on private versus academic practice, registration in the computer seminar, years in practice, participation in research activities, or prior computer experience. The authors concluded that physicians would be more accepting of computer systems that serve as a tool to aid in providing optimal patient care and less accepting of applications where the computer functions as a substitute for the physician.

When physicians ranked expectations for computers in the same survey, they expected that it was most likely that computer consultation systems would increase government control of physicians' practices, be blamed for ineffective treatment, increase the costs of care, and threaten personal and professional privacy. They felt that it would be least likely that systems would result in less efficient use of physician time, reduce the need for specialists and paraprofessionals, or require physicians to "think like computers." Academic physicians and residents, younger physicians, and those with computer experience had the most positive expectations for computer consultation programs. The survey questions in this study reflect early concerns about the "big brother" aspects of computers. This topic is hardly even mentioned in the current debate about computers, possibly because oversight of the quality, costs, and process of care has become a fact of life in today's health care delivery system.

In 1981, a survey about computer attitudes was mailed to a national sample of approximately 1,000 internists and otolaryngologists in academic and private practice and in residency training programs.(3) Ninety-two percent of the 276 respondents felt that a computer database would improve their access to information in the literature; 86 percent thought that access to a computer database would result in an improvement in their practice of medicine. Desirable capabilities of computer databases (in descending order of benefit) included literature summaries, patient registry, providing probability estimates of side effects of treatment, providing probability estimates of success of treatment, and providing probability estimates of a diagnosis. Some differences emerged in the rating of benefits among subgroups of respondents: academic physicians rated the capability to estimate probabilities higher than practicing physicians; otolaryngologists rated a computerized patient registry higher than internists. Overall, 76 percent of respondents stated that they would like to implement computers in their practice.

This study was the first designed to examine differences in attitudes toward computers between physicians of different specialties. Few differences in attitudes toward computers by specialty were uncovered, possibly because the categories of use included in the survey were broad enough to be generally applicable to both specialties.

A study of nurses' and social workers' attitudes toward computers was conducted at one rehabilitation hospital in the early 1980s.(4) The survey contained 14 statements about personal resistance to computers, eight statements about organizational resistance to computers, and three questions about experience with computers. Eighty percent of the respondents rated themselves as novice computer users. Ratings of computers in general were uniformly positive; 85 percent agreed that computers would offer benefits to their profession. As a group, nurses and social workers rated specific computer support to clinical practice lower than statements about computers in general. However, when examined separately, the nurses were positive about specific clinical applications, while social workers were negative.

A study conducted in the 1980s in a large Ohio teaching hospital was designed to evaluate nurses' perceptions of computers. Ninety percent of respondents felt that computers would increase their productivity and effectiveness; 80 percent felt that they personally would gain satisfaction from using computers; and 57 percent felt that they would be challenged rather than frustrated if they encountered problems using a computer. Less than 3 percent of the nurses wished computers would "never come." Older staff, those with more education, and those with prior computer experience had the most positive attitudes toward computers.(5)

In 1985, a survey was distributed to all 160 freshman, 130 juniors, and a sample of 200 faculty members at a U.S. medical school.(6) The survey contained 48 questions related to demographics, computer experience, attitudes toward computers, and recommendations for use of computers in medical education. Some of the aspects of computers that were rated positively (listed in descending order of the percentage of respondents agreeing with the statement) were: time for the physician-patient interaction, validity of patient information, enhanced assessment of hospital and clinic performance, timeliness of patient data, patient compliance with physician directions, quality of the patient-physician interaction, and not interfering with physicians' authority and power. However, more than half the respondents agreed that computers would negatively affect the confidentiality of the physician-patient interaction and the "personal touch."

Respondents' experience with and education in computers was not correlated with attitudes toward computer systems. Students consistently displayed more positive attitudes toward computers than faculty members. When asked if they had reservations about specific uses of computers, less than 10 percent of the total sample expressed strong reservations about computer use in general. There were no differences in attitudes among different medical specialists. Physicians with fewer than 20 years in practice were more positive about the benefits of computers in terms of use of the patients' time and the timeliness of data. Older faculty members had more concerns about the intrusion of computers into the medical decision process.

The contrast between this 1985 study and earlier findings is interesting in that physicians and medical students rated the ability to monitor performance as an important positive benefit of computers, whereas in some of the earlier studies the potential for oversight of the patient care process was perceived to be a negative implication. By 1985, it was clear that hospital, departmental, and individual performance would be reviewed by outside groups. Physicians may have felt the efficient, comprehensive review possible with computers was preferable to alternative manual review methods.

A study conducted in the mid-1980s compared nurses' attitudes in a hospital where computers were used for order entry and results retrieval, medication administration lists, and care planning with attitudes in another hospital without computers on the nursing units.(7) On a scale of 20 (least favorable) to 100 (most favorable), the mean score among users was 70 and the mean score among nonusers was 72. Users of computers were less likely to perceive the computer as a threat to job security, but nonusers had more positive attitudes about the capabilities of computers and the amount of time that would be freed up by using computers.

There was no difference between users and nonusers in attitudes toward legal ramifications of computer use, perception of nurses' willingness to use computers, and institutional benefits derived from computer use. There was no difference in attitudes based on age or years worked as a nurse. The authors speculated that the attitudes of computer users would be improved if the computer system was tailored to meeting the needs of nurses and if it were used more effectively.

In the late 1980s, a survey was used to compare the attitudes of nursing students and practicing nurses.(8) Both practicing nurses and nursing students had positive attitudes toward computers, but nursing students were more positive than practicing nurses, especially on survey items related to use of computers in patient care. There was no significant difference between the students and practicing nurses on items related to security or general attitudes toward computers.

At about the same time, another study of nursing attitudes toward computers was conducted in a district hospital in England.(9) The survey database was used to compare the responses of different subgroups of nurses. No difference in attitudes was found based on age of the respondent, length of total nursing or length of experience at the particular hospital, present computer experience, educational training, or type of ward (medical, surgical, or operating room).

Since it now seems clear that computers will be used in health care settings, assessing general attitudes toward computers is no longer a high priority. However, there may be new uses for detailed attitude surveys. The value of using attitudinal surveys to plan for optimal implementation of computer systems has been demonstrated by researchers at Intermountain Health Care.(10) A detailed pre-implementation survey was developed that contained questions about attitudes toward installation of the computer system, design of computer training, and priorities for computer support. The surveys were distributed to physicians and dentists, nurses, and other staff members prior to the installation of the HELP System at McKay-Dee Hospital.

The responses were analyzed to identify areas of general agreement and disagreement related to the implementation of the computer system. There was agreement about the need for hands-on training–the importance of making the system easy to use, having terminals accessible, ensuring continuous operation, and maintaining confidentiality of records–and the importance of involving users in implementation. Analysis of responses indicated that respondents who were most experienced with computers held stronger opinions about both the benefits and potential problems associated with automation. The responses of different types of staff were compared to identify discrepancies in automation priorities that might indicate potential conflicts during implementation. No such conflicts were found and the consensus on implementation priorities was communicated to the system developers.

Use of Computers by Physicians and Nurses

Starting in the 1980s patient care information systems (often with limited capabilities) were installed in a number of hospitals and ambulatory care clinics. This enabled researchers to investigate whether positive attitudes toward the concept of computers would be accompanied by widespread use of these systems by physicians and nurses.

Because no hospitals in the United States have converted to a totally automated medical record(11), manual charts are typically available as an alternative to the computer. Assuming that the paper chart can be found and the computer system can be accessed, physicians and nurses can choose between using the computer or the manual chart to retrieve patient information. In some hospitals with computer support to ordering, physicians are given the option of entering orders into a system directly or having them transcribed into the system by the nursing staff. Whenever computers are available as an option, the percentage of time the computer is chosen over the manual alternative is a good measure of acceptance of the computer system.

The most common use of computers by physicians is to retrieve patient results. Boston's Beth Israel Hospital examined the frequency of this use of a comprehensive patient care information system.(12) The hospital had an average daily census of 455 patients. During a 1-week study conducted in 1984, 818 different clinical providers (staff physicians, nurses, residents, and medical students) used the computer 16,768 times to look up patient results. Since traditional paper records were available, use of the computer was optional. About 75 percent of the uses of the system were related to inpatient care; the average number of look-ups per inpatient was four times each day. However, for 18 percent of the inpatients the system was not used to retrieve information during the week of the study. The most frequent use of the results retrievable capability was to obtain a consolidated summary of most recent results (used 6,972 times), then (in descending order of use) chemistry results, hematology results, radiology reports, demographics and visit history, microbiology, blood gases, surgical pathology reports, and, finally, outpatient pharmacy profiles (accessed 32 times during the week).

Eighty percent of providers who had used the system more than 10 times indicated in a user survey that they used the system "most of the time" to retrieve laboratory test results.(12)

In 1988, the study of use of the clinical computer system at Beth Israel Hospital was repeated.(13) Data were also obtained at the second teaching hospital that was using the same software. At Beth Israel Hospital, the total number of uses to look up inpatient information in 1988 was 27,729 per week (for 900 patients), an increase of almost 119 percent over the 1984 level. The relative frequency of computer use for different types of information did not differ markedly from 1984, and the most frequent use of the system still was to retrieve all the most recent patient results. There were 13,299 inquiries for 4,379 outpatients (three uses per patient), an increase of 324 percent from the level measured in 1984. A new capability for physicians to enter orders for electrocardiograms was used 174 times during the week. Data on use by type of staff indicate that residents used the system an average of 54 times per week to look up patient information for inpatients and outpatients, medical students 49 times per week, clinical fellows 29 times per week, nurses 16 times per week, and staff physicians 14 times per week.

At the second hospital using the system, 40,998 inquiries for clinical information about 1,306 inpatients occurred during the week of the study. At this hospital the most frequent use of the system was also to obtain an integrated display of the most recent results.

The authors of these studies expressed the opinion that system developers should not ask, "How can we get physicians to use computers?," because this was clearly achievable. Instead, they recommended that future developers ask, "How can we make computers more helpful?"–a question that is still applicable today.

The fact that well-designed patient care systems will be used by health care providers is also supported by research at Columbia Presbyterian Medical Center, a large (1,500-bed) teaching hospital.(14) The system at Columbia permits the user to review laboratory results; reports of electrocardiograms, electroencephalograms, radiology, pathology, and endoscopic procedures; and discharge summaries (as well as for electronic mail and other functions). A study of the use of that system by clinical staff showed that on an average weekday, 810 staff members used the system on 2,531 occasions to make about 5,400 inquiries of the clinical database. As shown in Figure 2-1, residents were the

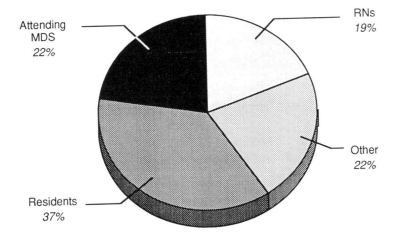

Figure 2-1. Distribution of the Use of Computerized Information Retrieval in an Inpatient Setting(14)

heaviest users of the computer. Usage of the system also varied by specialty. Eighty-three percent of attending physicians within the medicine department used the system at least once during the week-long study, whereas only 50 percent of the surgeons were system users.

A patient care system (3M HELP) installed at Rex Hospital provides capability for physicians to review or print patient lists, test results, procedure reports, medication lists, and demographic information. A 1990 survey of physicians indicated that 34 percent of the respondents used these features frequently and 42 percent never used them. Nonusers had concerns about ease of use and the time required to access information. The hospital responded by developing a new computerized Rounds Report that generated reports for a list of patients without the need to select items individually. The time period for reporting, the time sequencing of data, and the type of data included could be customized.

A 9-month study of use of the Rounds Report indicated it was used by 17 percent of the staff. The highest percentage of users were physicians in infectious disease, hematology/oncology, pulmonary, gynecology, and internal medicine. Sixty-two percent of the users requested customized reports; 94 percent preferred data in reverse chronological order; and 46 percent of the time reports were viewed only on the screen. Physicians tended to specify one report format and use it consistently. Heavy users were specialist consultants who were neither trained in system use nor involved in the development of the system. However, even among this group, the system was not used in preference to the chart on a daily basis.(15)

Most of the experience with patient care computers has been obtained in an inpatient setting. The ambulatory setting presents new challenges. Kaiser Permanente Mid-Atlantic States has equipped all physicians with personal computers with capabilities for retrieval of results, maintaining problem lists, accessing demographics, and recording progress notes. The system is used by physicians at 95 percent of all visits and two to three screens are reviewed per visit.(16)

With computerized records, the cost of computer storage increases proportionately with the volume of information in the record. In inpatient care, information often is stored only in paper format after a patient is discharged. This is not a viable option for outpatient care. However, if "old" data were used rarely, it might be possible to store old data offline in machine readable form, only retrieving the information when it is needed. The use of data more than 1 year old was examined at Pacific Medical Center, a group of large and small clinics in Seattle.(17) This center was using an integrated patient care information system supplied by PHAMIS with 5 years of data available in the computer on appointments, patient encounters, prescriptions, laboratory results, and radiology reports. The computer provided an alternative to the traditional paper record, so use of the system was optional.

Computer printouts of the current patient medication profile and printouts of test results were filed in each patient's paper record. Prior to a patient visit, the medical assistant often printed out summary data from the previous visit or a summary of information for a particular problem being followed. In addition, computer terminals were available in the clinics for physicians to use directly. Direct use of the system by providers was studied for 1 week to quantify use of the system for retrieval of information more than 1 year old. Seventy-two percent of the providers in the study used the terminals to retrieve information a total of 1,982 times during the study week (two uses per patient). For 17 percent of the patients, a laboratory result more than 1 year old was requested. Forty-four percent of these requests for "old" data were for information between 1 and 2 years old, 37 percent were for data 2 to 3 years old, and 19 percent for data more than 3 years old.

A survey was conducted to determine what actions providers would take if old data were not available to them on the computer. The most frequent responses were that they would pull the old paper chart or treat the patient with less information. However, more than 30 percent said they would order more tests, and some providers said they would maintain their own flow sheets if old data were not available on the computer system.

The results of this study indicate that taking data offline will be problematic. Providers frequently need to access old information, and in the outpatient environment where patient volumes are high, it will not be feasible to bring old data back from offline storage. The alternatives of having each provider create his or her own manual records, repeat tests, or treat without needed information are not attractive options.

It has always been recognized that designing systems that enable providers to *retrieve* information would be much simpler than designing efficient methods for *entry* of information. In 1978, a patient care computer system supplied by TDS was installed in a 1,000-bed teaching hospital and use of the system by physicians for ordering was studied.(18) Physicians had the option of entering medication orders into the system directly or having their handwritten orders sent to the pharmacy, where they were transcribed into the computer by a pharmacy technician. With either mode of data entry, the orders were available on the computer for nurses to use when charting which medications were administered.

Approximately 2,500 inpatient pharmacy orders were placed each day. During the first year of system use, the method of data entry for pharmacy orders was analyzed. At that time physicians were entering 70 percent of all prescriptions directly into the computer. When the study was repeated five years later, 98 percent of the orders were entered into the system directly by physicians.

The conventional wisdom in 1978 (and continuing to this day) is that physicians will resist assuming the task of entering orders into a computer system. Pharmacy orders are especially problematic to enter; the number of possible medications is large and, therefore, complex orders may require several screens. Once the drug is ordered, the dosage, route of administration, start date and time and end date and time all must be specified. The authors attribute success at this hospital to the implementation approach (providing an optional manual process, stationing pharmacy staff on the units during the first weeks of implementation to provide instruction and support) and to the value the physicians placed on having medication orders for their patients processed quickly.

Another teaching hospital (using the same computer system) had a quite different experience with direct physician order entry.(19) A study of use of the computers by physicians for order entry over a 6-week period documented a wide variation in use by specialty of the physician. The highest use was by cardiovascular surgeons or their physicians' assistants; they entered 13 percent of all orders directly into the computer. (This was the only specialty where assistants were allowed to enter orders.) The highest unassisted use was among neuro and orthopedic surgeons, who entered 5 percent of all orders directly. General surgeons, family practitioners, psychiatrists, neurologists, and urologists, entered less than 1 percent of their own orders. The study found that physicians who had developed personal order sets that enabled them to enter multiple orders were more likely to voluntarily use the computer system, as were physicians with positive attitudes toward computers.

At a third hospital implementing the same system, house staff became so frustrated with the time required to enter orders into the system that they instituted a "work action" where all orders were entered in free text–creating havoc in the receiving departments. The hospital instituted a series of actions to improve the ordering–the most effective was reported to be creation of order sets.(20)

In another hospital, house staff vocally opposed the task of entering orders into a computer system so they were provided with the alternative of having a medical student or an information systems staff member enter orders.(21) The transcription service was available from 10 a.m. to 6 p.m. Physicians elected to use transcription for only 16 percent of the orders entered when the service was available. However, it is likely that the transcription service did not coincide with peak ordering times (after morning rounds). The authors suggested that physicians may not have trusted medical students and information systems staff to transcribe the orders properly.

The mixed success documented in studies of physician ordering seems to reflect market experience. Some of the hospitals that implemented physician ordering have achieved total compliance. Others encountered strong opposition. There are now more success stories, probably due to improved designs that minimize the time cost of ordering by computer and integrate ordering with other uses of the computer.(22)

Of course, to create a complete record of patient care will require that other text information in addition to orders be entered into the computer. When part of the general medicine/primary care clinic at Beth Israel Hospital in Boston was moved to a site outside the hospital, outpatient medical records for those patients were also moved off site. Physicians in the remote clinic were offered a computer system to use in entering and maintaining problem lists, medication lists, health promotions screening sheets, flow sheets, and progress notes.(23) The main objective for computerization was to increase access at the hospital to clinical information about patients treated at the off-site clinic. Eighteen months later, the capability for entering clinic documentation was expanded to the general medicine and primary care clinics at the hospital.

When utilization of different capabilities was examined after 2 years of use at the remote site, 68 percent of the patients had problem lists and 70 percent had medication lists on the computer. At the main clinic, where the system had been in use for only three months, 22 percent of the patients had problem lists and 29 percent had medication lists on the system. Three of 11 staff physicians and 19 of 51 residents at the main clinic had never used the system to enter information, and only one staff physician and eight residents used the computer system to record all problems and medications. As shown in Figure 2-2, the maintenance of the computerized problem and medication lists varied among different types of staff. Interns and nurse practitioners used computerized documentation more than residents and staff physicians

A follow-up report of 4 years of experience indicated that it took about 6 months of system use for physicians to experience time savings from use of the computer-based encounter reports and to become enthusiastic about system use. An electronic note feature was added to the system in response to physicians' demands. A survey of use indicated the interns and residents voluntarily type in notes for about half of all patient encounters.(24)

An ambulatory care clinic at the University of Nebraska Hospital conducted a trial using a computer system to document telephone encounters.(25) The objective was to increase the number of telephone encounters that were documented. Before automation, none of these calls was documented. A review of 56 telephone encounters revealed that using the computer, nurses documented

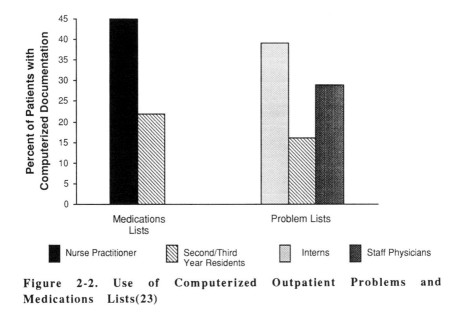

Figure 2-2. Use of Computerized Outpatient Problems and Medications Lists(23)

case management decisions 65 percent of the time. However, when patients called for information (e.g., test results, procedure preparations) less than 5 percent of the encounters were documented in the computer. This may indicate that the future value of the information is a factor that motivates patient care staff to use computer systems to document care.

These studies document that voluntary physician use of computers was attractive to some providers and not to others. This study reinforces the need to better understand differences among voluntary computer users, and to identify whether system design or educational changes might increase the voluntary use of computers–especially for data entry.

One long-held expectation for computers is that they would go beyond serving as input and output devices for patient information and assist in physician decision making. However, clinical decision support capabilities have been absent in most commercial systems. The HELP system is one commercial product that does contain decision aids. A 16-month study of use of the HELP patient care computer system at LDS Hospital in Salt Lake City showed that for 88,500 medication orders entered for 13,727 patients, the computer generated 690 alerts.(26) The most common alert related to conflicting laboratory data (45 percent of alerts), followed by drug interactions (30 percent), drug allergies (16 percent), and dosage (7 percent). Another study at the same institution documented that computerized drug alerts were generated for between 8 and 9 percent of all patients. For 1.8 percent of patients, the alerts warned of situations that were considered to be life threatening. Physicians complied with computer-generated medication alerts 99 percent of the time.

Direct entry of orders by physicians is a necessary prerequisite to providing direct, timely feedback to influence ordering patterns, and complete documentation of encounters will be essential if computers are used for decision support. As was discussed previously, it has been demonstrated that such feedback can both reduce the number of tests ordered and increase compliance with protocols for care. This group of studies indicates that offering physicians the option of voluntary use of computer systems results in a wide range of acceptance. A review of past studies raises some interesting questions about design of the software to support ordering, system performance (response time, downtime, etc.), access to terminals, satisfaction with alternatives to computer entry, or other factors that influence the extent to which physicians will voluntarily enter orders into a computer system.

Several investigations have speculated that characteristics of the users also influence whether or not a patient care system will be used. Information on the correlation of computer use with age of the attending physician was obtained in an evaluation of the use of clinical information system at Columbia Presbyterian Medical Center for 1 year (1992).(27) Sixty-one percent of attending physicians voluntarily used the system during the year. Age explained only 3 percent of the variance in usage. For physicians who admitted more than 50 patients during the year, 100 percent of physicians younger than 32 used the system, and 91 percent of attending physicians who were between 63 and 72 years old were users.

Usage rates by physicians between ages 33 and 62 were lower than those for physicians over 63 or under 32. The lowest usage rates (69 percent) were among physicians between 53 and 62 years of age. The highest usage of the system was among physicians in medicine (mean of 14.7 uses per case); neurology (7.1 uses per case); pediatrics (3.5 uses per case) and surgery (3.3 uses per case). Lowest usage was in OB/GYN, neurosurgery, otolaryngology, and orthopedic surgery (0.8 to 1.2 uses per case). There was significant variation in usage both among different specialties and within a specialty.

The authors speculate that usage is influenced by the value provided by the system. We have found similar patterns of usage by age and specialty in our research, and we have concluded that *value to the user* is the key driver of use. We suspect that the difference in use by age may be due to the different roles of older versus younger physicians and that difference in use by specialty is related to the information intensity and information dependence of each specialty.

Satisfaction with Clinical Computers

Satisfaction is the most common measure of acceptance of computers, probably because of the ease with which satisfaction information can be collected. Two types of satisfaction studies have been conducted. Some studies report data on overall satisfaction, typically as part of a related study on computer experience. The second type of satisfaction study provides detailed information on satisfaction with specific uses of a computer system, specific features, or specific benefits. Although most of these detailed studies pose their questions in terms of satisfaction, they are really intended to rate the system's capabilities and uses. The surveys of overall satisfaction are only useful in justifying an investment or pointing out that further development is needed. However, detailed satisfaction studies can provide information on capabilities and design features that are attractive or unattractive to different groups of users.

What many consider to be the landmark study of patient care information systems was conducted at El Camino Hospital in 1971. This computer was used for entering orders, retrieving results, and charting medications for inpatients.(28) Initially, physicians were required to enter their orders into the system; within a few months, order entry was made voluntary for physicians. Twenty expectations for the system had been identified by interviewing physicians before the system was installed. Two years after the system's installation, physicians were surveyed to determine if the system had met their expectations. More than 50 percent of physicians reported that their expectations had been met or exceeded in terms of decreased frequency of medication errors, control of scheduled medications that are actually given, and reduced ambiguity of orders. More than 75 percent of physicians reported that their expectations for providing information in a more convenient and accessible form, and for improved quality of patient care had *not* been met. When asked to compare prior manual and computer-supported operations, 60 percent felt that retrieving current orders was better with the computer and 53 percent felt that having test data available in a reasonable amount of time was better. Eighty percent felt that handling printed reports was worse with the computer, and between 50 and 60 percent felt several other aspects of information management had declined: locating and assimilating nurses' narrative information, locating printed laboratory results in the chart, and assessing patient data.

At the same hospital, nurses' satisfaction was also assessed. More than 75 percent of all respondents agreed that the admission, discharge, and transfer processes had improved with computer support; and over 50 percent agreed that the ward clerks had more responsibility, the unit was better organized, and that there had been an improvement in care planning. However, 39 percent disagreed with statements that downtime did not interfere with nursing care and that the quality of patient care had increased. More than 50 percent of nurses agreed that, with the computer system, medications were administered and charted more efficiently, the shift report was more complete, doctor's orders were easier to read, laboratory results were easier to interpret, and that charting patient care was easier. However, 92 percent also agreed that an excessive amount of paper was generated with the system.

While this particular study is quite old and the system that was evaluated in 1973 has been replaced with a newer version, the study results do indicate the advantage of obtaining detailed satisfaction data in evaluations of computer systems. These data permit many aspects of computer use (usefulness of functions and system design features) to be evaluated, and allow the manual and computer operations to be compared. For example, the results of this study pointed to formatting, printing, and filing of paper output from the system as aspects of system design that needed improvement, and system downtime and response time as areas where technical performance was suboptimal.

In one study of a clinical computer system discussed earlier(12), nurses and physicians who had used the system more than 10 times received an online survey about their satisfaction. Eighty-nine percent of respondents rated the system as "very helpful" (the highest rating on a five-point Likert scale). The authors note that ratings by staff physicians, house officers, nurses, and medical students were similar.

The most information-dependent area of a hospital is probably the intensive care unit. A survey conducted of physicians' and nurses' satisfaction with information before and after a computer system was installed in an intensive care unit indicated that both physicians and nurses were neutral or positive about the changes brought about by the computer system.(29) Nurses' satisfaction with the computer was measured after 2 days and 2 months of use, and no significant differences were found between the two time periods. Younger, less-experienced nurses had more positive attitudes toward the computer system; the sample was too small to examine the responses of physicians by age group.

It is interesting to note that while physicians' and nurses' ratings of their overall satisfaction with the computer were almost identical, physicians were less satisfied than nurses with specific aspects of the system. For example, 90 percent of nurses reported that the computer made the task of recording fluid input and output easier, while only 44 percent of physicians rated the computer as creating improvement in this area. The researchers hypothesized that the screens used by physicians to retrieve this information were not well designed. Also, while most tasks were rated as enhanced with the computer system, some items, such as obtaining temperature and pulse information, were rated as better under the manual system. This type of detailed satisfaction data enabled the system developers to identify specific targets for improving the design of the system.

Most studies have measured satisfaction with a computer system at one point in time. In the late 1980s, nurses' attitudes toward computers were measured just before and 3 and 6 months after the introduction of a computer system. Acceptance was measured by the nurses' self-assessment of their willingness to use computers for nine different activities (e.g., enter orders, use as a reference, generate care plans). There was no significant difference in willingness to use computers at different points in time. Nurses were also asked about their concerns about computers. The main concern expressed was that the computer would take time away from direct patient care. This concern decreased (but did not disappear) during the time frame of the study. Nurses' willingness to use the computer was not affected by age, education, length of time in health care, or prior computer experience.(30)

A survey of 300 physicians who used a comprehensive computer system at LDS Hospital in Salt Lake City was conducted in the spring of 1989. The survey results related to pharmacy services have been published.(26) On a scale of 1 to 5, where 5 was the most positive response, alerts related to life-threatening situations were rated as 4.63 in importance and generating pharmacy alerts at the time of order entry was rated 4.35. When asked about future applications, expansion of laboratory alerts was the highest priority, followed by access to a pharmacy knowledge base. Though these results relate to a very specific application of computers, they do illustrate the value of having detailed satisfaction data to guide system design.

User satisfaction with computer systems has also been studied in outpatient settings. A 1975 study of computer-based ambulatory records systems included nine different sites.(31) At eight sites, the researchers administered a survey instrument. A total of 58 surveys were returned (for several sites there were only two respondents). The survey revealed an overall sightly positive attitude toward automated medical record systems among physician users. The results were skewed by one site that contributed about 50 percent of the surveys in the database and where attitudes were unusually negative.

An evaluation of the implementation of the COSTAR patient record system at a large HMO included an assessment of the acceptability of the system to providers. Fifty-eight of the 85 physicians and nurse clinicians preferred or strongly preferred delivering patient care with the computer and only one provider strongly preferred the manual system.(32)

Staff satisfaction was tracked before, immediately after, and 18 months after the COSTAR medical record system was installed at University of Nebraska clinics. A controlled trial was conducted where the COSTAR system was used for a selected set of visits, and paper records for the remainder. Data were analyzed for 15 staff who completed all three questionnaires. At all periods, the staff preferred the following attributes of the COSTAR medical record: finding the record, finding the most recent encounter, readability, time to find information, time spent answering billing questions, handling phone calls, and managing prescription refills. They preferred the paper medical record only for reviewing the hospitalization summaries, which were not available in the COSTAR system.(33)

Another satisfaction study provides detailed information about physicians' satisfaction with a computer system to support outpatient care.(34) Satisfaction data for the study were collected in a general medicine clinic at a Veterans Administration System hospital after a new computer system was installed. The new computer system was developed at Regenstrief Institute and, therefore, is referred to as the Regenstrief System. It was used to link together separate computer systems in the laboratory, pharmacy, and patient appointment scheduling so that physicians could obtain integrated information about patients. Encounter reports were also transcribed into the new system.

The physicians were asked to provide ratings of their opinions about the new system (Regenstrief interfaced to the departmental systems), versus the old departmental systems alone. For 14 of 15 specific items, physicians reported higher satisfaction with the new integrated system. Selected results are provided in Table 2-1. The areas of greatest improvement were for items related to prescription information and contribution of the system to the efficiency of care delivery. The only item not rated as better with the new system was access to information from other clinics.

The detailed nature of the questions in this survey permits different aspects of the system uses to be compared; this type of information would be useful in helping guide future design. These results suggest that having medication profiles online provides a significant benefit in outpatient care. However, the limited scope of the study (one general medicine clinic) and the fact that providers were asked to rate both the old and new systems at the same time–after the experimental system was installed–raise some concern about bias.

A study of nurses' reactions to a system for documenting telephone encounters in an ambulatory care clinic also showed positive attitudes.(25) Nurses agreed with a statement about positive changes due to the computer and disagreed that patients were uncomfortable when they typed information into the system and that it would be better to go back to keeping manual records. On a scale where 5 represented a strong preference for using the computer and 1 a strong preference for paper records, the following items all scored above 4: ability to find records, organization and legibility of records, and availability of information on current problems and medications. The highest rated benefits of

Table 2-1. Difference in Satisfaction Before vs. After
Availability of Integrated Outpatient Information

Aspect of System Use	Mean Likert Value
Ease of locating information	+2.1
Organization of information	+2.3
Accuracy of information	+2.2
Improvement of efficiency	+2.5
Prescription profiles, easy to use	+2.7
Time spent with patients	+1.8
Avoidance of mistakes`	+1.8
Overall satisfaction with the system	+2.0

the system were assistance in communicating with other staff, efficiency of handling prescription refills, and recording information from telephone calls.

Summary

It seems clear that patient care information systems have been accepted by users in many settings, but that acceptance is not universal. If we intend to use computer-based records systems to manage patient care across a continuum of care, systems must be accepted by all those who provide direct patient care. The needs of physicians and nurses are probably very different because they make different types of decisions in different settings. Information priorities will likely vary by specialty. Requirements for inpatient care, where a large quantity of information must be obtained and evaluated in a short period of time, are quite different from the needs in outpatient care, where less information needs to be tracked over longer periods of time. In inpatient care, clerical staff, nurses, and physicians typically share the responsibility for managing information, whereas in outpatient care, the physician may have no support staff available to track down missing information. Therefore, understanding acceptance of computer-based medical record systems will require assessing the views of many different users in many different settings.

Detailed attitude and satisfaction data have been shown to be helpful in challenging some commonly held beliefs about acceptance of systems, in improving their design, and in planning for implementation. Based on the current state of the art in development and use of computers, and the need to gain the benefits that computer-based systems can offer, one important research question is:

- What features and functions of computer systems are currently acceptable for clinical use, and what improvements are needed to increase the value of these systems?

Answering this question requires detailed information on acceptance of specific features and functions in a wide variety of settings, and information on when manual systems are currently preferred. In the following chapters we will present study results and experience designed to answer questions about the value of specific system features and functions, and other critical success factors for implementing patient care information systems.

References

1. Zoltan-Ford E, Chapanis A. What do professional persons think about computers? Behavior and Information Technology 1982;1:55-68.
2. Teach RI, Shortliffe E. Analysis of physician attitudes regarding computer-based clinical consultation systems. Computers in Biomedical Research 1981;14:542-558.
3. Singer J, Sacks HS, Lucente F, Chalmers TC. Physician attitudes toward applications of computer database systems. Journal of the American Medical Association 1983;249:1610-1614.
4. Mandell SF. Resistance to computerization. Journal of Medical Systems 1987;11:311-318.
5. Krampf S, Robinson S. Managing nurses' attitudes toward computers. Nursing Management July 1984;15:29-34
6. Knapp RG, Miller MC, Levine J. Experience with and attitudes toward computers in medicine of students and clinical faculty members at one school. Journal of Medical Education 1987;62:344-346.
7. Bomgartz, C. Computer-oriented patient care. Computers in Nursing 1988; 6;204-210.
8. Schwirian PM, Malone JA, Stone VJ, Nunley B, Francisco T. Computers in nursing practice; a comparison of the attitudes of nurses and nursing students. Computers in Nursing 1989;7:168-177.
9. Sultana N. Nurses' attitudes towards computerization in clinical practice. Journal of Advanced Nursing 1990;15:696-702.
10. Lundsgaarde HP, Gardner RM, Menlove RL. Using attitudinal questionnaires to achieve benefits optimization. Proceedings of the 14th Annual SCAMC. IEEE Computer Society Press, 1989;703-707.
11. Dick RS and Steen E. The Computer-based patient record: an essential technology for health care. National Academy Press, 1991.
12. Bleich HL, Beckley RF, Horowitz GL, et al. Clinical computing in a teaching hospital. New England Journal of Medicine 1985;312:756-764.

13. Safran C, Slack W, Bleich H. Role of computing in patient care in two hospitals. M.D. Computing 1989;6:1,2,143-148.
14. Hendrickson G, Anderson RK, Clayton PD. The integrated academic information management system at Columbia Presbyterian Medical Center. M.D. Computing 1992;9:35-42.
15. Michael P. Physician-directed software design: the role of utilization statistics and user input in enhancing HELP results review capabilities. Proceeding of the 17th Annual SCAMC, IEEE Computer Society Press, 1993;107-111.
16. Dewey JB, Manning P, Brandt S. Acceptance of direct physician access to a computer-based patient record in a managed care setting. Proceedings of the 17th Annual SCAMC, IEEE Computer Society Press, 1993;79-83.
17. Gleser M, and Mathews M. Clinical value of a long term database: a study of providers at Pacific Medical Center. Presentation at the 15th Annual SCAMC 1992.
18. Schroeder C, Pierpach P. Direct order entry by physicians in a computerized hospital information system. American Journal of Hospital Pharmacy 1986;43:355-359.
19. Anderson JG, Jay S, Schweer HM, Anderson MM. Perceptions of the impact of computers in medical practice and physician use of a hospital information system. Proceedings of the 5th Annual SCAMC 1985;565-569.
20. Massaro TA. Introduction physician order entry at a major academic medical center: impact on organizational culture and behavior. Academic Medicine 1993;68:20-24.
21. Spillane MJ, McLaughlin MB, Ellis KK, Montgomery WL, Dziuban S. Direct physician order entry and integration: potential pitfalls. Proceedings of the 14th Annual SCAMC; IEEE Computer Society Press, 1990;774-778.
22. Teich JM, Spurr CD, Flammini SJ, Schiz J, Beckley RF, Hurley JF, Aranow M, Glaser P. Response to a trial of physician-based inpatient order entry. Proceedings of the 17th Annual SCAMC, IEEE Computer Society Press, 1993;316-320.
23. Safran C, Rury C, Rind DM, Taylor WC. A computer-based outpatient medical record for a teaching hospital. M.D. Computing 1991;8:291-299.
24. Rind DM, Safran C. Real and imagined barriers to an electronic medical record. Proceedings of the 17th SCAMC, IEEE Computer Society Press, 1994;74-78.
25. Stoupa R, Campbell J. Documentation of ambulatory care rendered by telephone: use of a computerized nursing model. Proceedings of the 14th Annual SCAMC. IEEE Computer Society Press, 1990;890-893.
26. Gardner R. Assessing the effectiveness of a computerized pharmacy system. Proceedings of the 14th Annual SCAMC. IEEE Computer Society Press, 1990;668-672.

27. Clayton PD, Pulver GE, Hill CL. Physician use of computers: is age or value the predominate factor? Proceedings of the 17th Annual SCAMC. IEEE Computer Society Press, 1994;301-305.

28. Battelle Memorial Institute. Evaluation of the implementation of a medical information system in a general community hospital. Arlington,VA:NTIS, 1973.

29. Gilhooly KJ, Logie R, Ross D, Ramayya P, Green C. Users' perceptions of a computerized information system in intensive care (ABICUS) on introduction and after 2 months use. International Journal of Clinical Monitoring and Computing 1991;8:101-106.

30. Feeney S, Donovan A. Changes in attitudes toward computers during implementation. Proceedings of the 13th Annual SCAMC, IEEE Computer Society Press, 1989:807-808.

31. Henley RR, Wiederhold G. An analysis of automated ambulatory medical records systems. Springfield, VA:NTIS, 1975.

32. Barnett GO. Computer-stored ambulatory record (COSTAR). Springfield,VA:NTIS 1976.

33. Campbell JR, Seelig CB, Wigton RS, Givner N, Patil K, Tape TG. Clinic function and computerized ambulatory records: a concurrent study with conventional records. Proceedings of the 12th Annual SCAMC. IEEE Computer Society Press, 1988;745-748.

34. Martin DK. Making the connection: the VA Regenstrief project. M.D. Computing 1992;9:91-96.

3
Physicians' and Nurses' Satisfaction with Patient Care Information Systems: Two Case Studies

Erica L. Drazen

Computer systems that process patient care information fall into three categories: departmental systems that automate patient data from areas such as pharmacy, laboratory, or radiology; dedicated systems that support patient care documentation processes (typically focused on nursing documentation); and integrated patient care information systems. The first category of support involves automation of specific types of patient data, such as laboratory results, radiology orders, ECG reports, and medication orders. Although these systems are often located within the responsible departments, terminals are sometimes located on the patient care floors for nurses and physicians to use in looking up patient information. Departmental systems have separate databases: one contains pharmacy information, another radiology information. In 1990, 43 percent of all U.S. hospitals had computer systems within their laboratory departments and 57 percent had computer systems within their pharmacy departments.(1)

Some patient care documentation systems are accessed at the bedside and used for functions such as recording the nursing history and the assessment of the patient, documenting the plan of care, and charting that the planned care has been delivered. Although most of these systems are used mainly by nursing staff, bedside documentation systems installed in intensive care areas are also used by physicians. About 150 hospitals in the United States have bedside systems installed; many more have centralized nursing documentation systems.(2)

The third type of information system to support patient care integrates patient information in a single database so that information can be accessed from many locations in an integrated form. The user can view information by patient rather than by the source of the data and can enter orders or documentation relative to any aspect of the patient's care. Today, integrated patient care information systems typically do not contain the full text portions of the medical record, nor do they feature the graphics and images that would be part of a totally computer-based patient record. However, integrated patient care information systems are closest to providing the information needed to truly manage patient care.

As discussed in Chapter 2, the results of research on acceptance, and research and market data on use of systems indicate that physicians and nurses do not resist the concept of computers. However, very few detailed studies indicate what type of computer support is needed, which functions nurses and physicians find most beneficial to automate, and where current systems fall short. In addition to information on benefits of computer support (discussed in Chapter 1) to set priorities for the future and learn how to improve all systems, research must also examine acceptance of specific computer-based applications, and satisfaction with different system designs and features.

Introduction to the Setting

In this chapter we will report on two case studies that provide detailed information on caregivers' information satisfaction with clinical departmental systems and patient care information systems. The information for the case studies was obtained from research performed by Arthur D. Little staff in Department of Defense (DoD) hospitals.(3) At the end of the chapter, we will compare the findings from these case studies with the results of research conducted in other settings.

The DoD hospitals provide an ideal setting for this research since in many respects the health care delivery model now in place in the DoD is representative of the future civilian care delivery system. The DoD provides comprehensive inpatient and outpatient care to active-duty and retired military personnel and their families. The population served reflects the full range of ages and diseases that would be seen in civilian settings and care is provided across the continuum of inpatient and outpatient settings.

Because active-duty physicians and nurses typically serve a minimum of 3 and a maximum of 20 years in the military as a group, they are younger than their civilian counterparts. These younger staff are typical of the computer experience and professional training that will be characteristic of the care providers of tomorrow. The settings represented in the case study include integrated, geographically dispersed care delivery systems; small community hospitals; and large teaching hospitals. The study hospitals were quite representative of the range of U.S. hospitals in terms of inpatient workload (average bed size of 252 beds compared with U.S. average for acute care general hospitals of 172 beds).(1) They have much higher outpatient volumes than a civilian hospital of similar size (350,000 visits per year compared with an average U.S. hospital volume of 55,000 visits per year).(4) In this respect they are probably representative of the ambulatory care focus of health care delivery systems in the future.

Care within the DoD is provided free of charge to all eligible patients. The DoD hospitals receive a fixed budget covering all inpatient and outpatient care for the population they serve. Most physicians are on salary. Therefore, in terms of financial incentives and billing paperwork, the DoD is also a good proxy for the future civilian delivery system.

One other advantage of the study setting is that the DoD made a decision to invest in a comprehensive evaluation and was willing to share the results–both benefits received and lessons learned–to advance our knowledge about acceptance of patient care computers. It is hoped that this willingness to invest in evaluation and share the results will also be a model for the future.

These case studies involved comparisons of 14 hospitals before and after an integrated patient care information system was installed in a subset of these hospitals. In their baseline state, the hospitals had a mix of departmental systems in their pharmacies and laboratories. Therefore, it was possible to examine both the impact of departmental systems and the effect of replacing these systems with an integrated patient care information system.

Introduction to the Computer Systems

The laboratory and pharmacy department systems installed in the study hospitals were all based on commercially available products that also were used in civilian hospitals. They offered capabilities that are quite typical of the systems currently installed in hospitals throughout the United States. The laboratory system supported entry of orders in all sections of the clinical laboratory; work scheduling; interface with analytic instruments; departmental reporting; and reporting of test results. In four of the six hospitals with laboratory department computers, a terminal was available in a central location in high-use patient care areas to permit look up of test status and laboratory results.

The pharmacy system was also a commercial product and provided a standard level of support within the pharmacy department: entry of orders, maintaining patient medication profiles, generating labels, and producing departmental reports. Access to the pharmacy system was available in patient care areas at only one site.

The integrated computer system that was installed in a subset of the hospitals in the case study is called the Composite Health Care System (CHCS). The system was developed by Science Applications International Corporation (SAIC) based on the software that had been developed and installed in Veterans Affairs hospitals. The CHCS is an integrated system that was designed to initially support patient registration; inpatient admission, discharge, and transfer; outpatient appointment booking and history of visits; ordering and reporting results of diagnostic tests for inpatients and outpatients; ordering diets for inpatients; and ordering medications for inpatients and outpatients. Orders could be entered either individually or using order sets that could be tailored to the patients' diagnosis or the physician's preferences. Terminals were available in all inpatient care areas; in outpatient clinics, a terminal was located in the physician's office or exam room. Terminals were also available in staff lounges and other common areas.

All laboratory, radiology, and medication orders for outpatients were entered into the CHCS system by the outpatient physician. Orders for inpatients were entered directly into the computer by physicians or transcribed into the system by staff from the nursing or ancillary departments. Results were distributed to terminals in patient care areas and abnormal results were flagged. During the ordering process, information about drug allergies, drug or radiology test duplicates, and drug overlaps and interactions was provided to the user who could decide whether to override the warning. For outpatients, the system maintained a medication profile; medications ordered but not picked up in the pharmacy could be tracked. The CHCS also contained an electronic mail system that was used extensively for official hospital-wide communication, electronic meetings, and for staff to send messages to each other.

At the time of the study, the CHCS did not store or transmit images, nor was it used to store textual data such as history and physical exam, consult reports or progress notes, nursing assessment, or care plans. The system was only used in one study hospital to chart medications and nursing treatments. At this site, the system was also used by physicians to directly enter all orders for inpatients. In all sites, a traditional paper chart was still maintained and was available for use by physicians and nurses.

Introduction to the Study Design for the Departmental Computer Case Study

Since the intent of the DoD was to have physicians and nurses use the new CHCS system directly–eventually replacing the paper record–the satisfaction of physicians and nurses was one of the key measures used to evaluate the system. The primary study was designed to compare physicians' and nurses' satisfaction with information to support patient care before and after the CHCS system was installed. In order to adjust for other changes in operations that might occur between the before and after studies, parallel data collection was conducted at three control sites that would not receive the CHCS.

The baseline (pre-CHCS) satisfaction surveys were distributed at 11 hospitals scheduled to receive the CHCS system and at the three control hospitals. Since each of these hospitals had different departmental systems installed, they provided the data to compare physicians' and nurses' satisfaction at sites with and without support for laboratory and pharmacy information.

The satisfaction surveys contained detailed questions about satisfaction with different aspects of information (quality, accessibility, timeliness), types of information (laboratory, pharmacy, radiology), and different information tasks (ordering tests, receiving warning messages, retrieving results). Each survey also contained questions that were unrelated to information to be used in adjusting for general attitudes at each hospital during the study periods.

Because of the size of the database, the survey responses could also be used to compare the reactions to the systems among physicians in different specialties and settings, nurses in different areas of the hospital, and among staff of different ages.

Physicians' and Nurses' Satisfaction with Pharmacy and Laboratory Departmental Systems

In our search of the literature (summarized in Chapter 2) we could find no studies that examined the impact of departmental computer systems on physicians' and nurses' satisfaction. This is a bit puzzling since these systems have often been justified based on the improved level of information services provided to direct caregivers. Since we had obtained data on physicians' and nurses' satisfaction at 14 hospitals, some with and some without computer systems in the laboratory and pharmacy, we examined these data to see the effect of a departmental computer on satisfaction. All 14 hospitals were included in the examination of laboratory and pharmacy systems, categorized either as a site with or without the relevant departmental automation.

Methodology

The data collected in this case study were analyzed to answer the question: Do physicians and nurses at hospitals with and without computer systems in the pharmacy and laboratory have different levels of satisfaction with related clinical information to support patient care?

Data on nurses' and physicians' satisfaction were collected using a paper survey. The nursing survey contained 17 questions about satisfaction with inpatient information, 14 general satisfaction questions that were not related to information, and one summary question about satisfaction with overall practice. The physicians' survey contained 18 questions related to outpatient information, 19 questions related to inpatient information, 19 general satisfaction questions unrelated to information, and two summary information questions. Both surveys included questions eliciting demographic information about the respondent. The questions dealt with all types of patient care information; therefore, only a subset of questions was relevant to the study of computers within pharmacy and laboratory departments.

Surveys used to assess satisfaction with laboratory and pharmacy systems were distributed through the internal hospital mail in the fall of 1988 through the spring of 1989. All nurses who delivered direct care for inpatients (not administrators) and who were registered nurses or had higher degrees in nursing received the nursing survey. All physicians, physicians assistants, and nurse practitioners who provided direct patient care for inpatients or outpatients received the "physician" survey. Sixty-six percent of the survey respondents to the physician survey were staff physicians, 24 percent were resident physicians, and 10 percent were other types of providers. Before data analysis began, the completed surveys were reviewed for quality; surveys that were returned blank or where demographic information indicated the respondent did not meet study criteria were eliminated.

The final database used to assess the effect of departmental systems included 1,119 nurses and 1,300 physicians from 14 sites. The overall survey response rate was 70 percent for nurses and 68 percent for physicians.

Responses to individual satisfaction questions were grouped together into satisfaction factors to facilitate the analysis. The factors that were created using a principal components factor analysis grouped questions with similar response patterns together. For nurses three information factors related to laboratory and pharmacy information were identified, and for physicians two outpatient information factors and two inpatient information factors related to laboratory information and medication information were created. The factors and survey items comprising each factor are shown in Table 3-1. In all of the analyses, respondents were dropped if they were missing more than 10 percent of the items making up a factor. The reliability of factors was evaluated using the Spearman-Brown measure of effective reliability (a measure of the intercorrelation among the items in each factor, adjusted for the number of items in the factor). Reliability of the factors ranged from 0.62 to 0.86.

Comparisons were made using analysis of variance (ANOVA) techniques, with the individual respondent as the unit of analysis. Initially, the effects of departmental computers were assessed using one-way ANOVA, with presence or absence of a specific departmental computer as the independent variable. Since we recognized that some variability in satisfaction with information might stem from differences in overall satisfaction at sites with and without departmental computers, the response to one survey question: "Overall, how satisfied are you with your practice at (name of the hospital)?" was used as a covariate to adjust for differences in general satisfaction levels. Inclusion of the general satisfaction question as a covariate enhanced our ability to isolate the effect of the departmental computer systems from other site and respondent effects.

The ANOVA was repeated with the following additional covariates for nursing: work location (general or critical care unit), age of respondent (30 and under, 31-40, and over 41), and facility size. The covariates were for physicians: clinic type (primary care or specialty), medical specialty of the provider, age of respondent, and facility size. When factors related to satisfaction with outpatient information were examined, facilities were grouped into four size ranges based on the number of outpatient visits: small (under 250,000 per year), medium (250,000-350,000), large (350,000-450,000), and very large (over 450,000). For factors related to inpatient information, facilities were grouped into three size

Table 3-1. Satisfaction Factors Used in the Departmental Automation Case Study

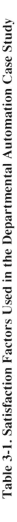

Nursing Satisfaction
Laboratory Results (Nurses)

- The process for notifying providers about abnormal laboratory diagnostic results
- Time you spend locating laboratory test results

Laboratory Turnaround (Nurses)

- Turnaround time for return of STAT laboratory test results
- Turnaround time for return of routine laboratory test results

Medication Information (Nurses)

- Completeness of information on medication administration records
- Accuracy of medication administration records in inpatient records

Physician Satisfaction with Outpatient Information

Medication Information for Outpatients (Physicians)

- Availability of outpatient medication profiles
- Completeness of outpatient medication profiles
- Availability of information on medication allergies

Laboratory Information for Outpatients (Physicians)

- Accuracy of test results
- Turnaround time for STAT laboratory test results
- Turnaround time for routine laboratory test results
- The process for notifying you about abnormal laboratory test result

Physician Satisfaction with Inpatient Information

Laboratory Information for Inpatients (Physicians)

- Turnaround time for STAT laboratory test results
- Turnaround time for routine laboratory test results
- Accuracy of test results in inpatient records
- The process for notifying you about abnormal laboratory results
- Medication information for inpatients (physicians)
- Medication information for inpatients
- Availability of information on medication allergies
- Completeness of information on patient's medication administration records
- Timeliness of information on medication administration records
- Accuracy of medication administration records in inpatient record

ranges according to the number of inpatient days of care provided per year: small (under 50,000 days); medium (50,000-100,000 days); and large (over 100,000 days).

Results

All results cited are mean Likert values for the factor, where the scale is from very dissatisfied (1) to very satisfied (5); 3 equals a neutral response. Throughout the discussion of results, the phrase *statistically significant result* means that a two-tailed test indicated that the result was significant at least at the 0.05 level. The numbers of respondents are approximate, since various numbers of respondents were dropped in each comparison.

Information Satisfaction Associated with Laboratory Computers

Satisfaction levels of approximately 710 inpatient nurses in six hospitals with laboratory computers were compared with responses from approximately 403 nurses in eight hospitals without laboratory systems. The effects of the laboratory computer on the laboratory results satisfaction factor and laboratory turnaround satisfaction factor were examined. Results are shown in Table 3-2. There was no significant difference in nurses' satisfaction with laboratory turnaround time at sites with and without laboratory computers. At sites with a laboratory computer, satisfaction with laboratory results was slightly higher. The laboratory results factor contained two items: the process for notifying providers about abnormal results and the time spent looking for laboratory results. No statistically significant differences in satisfaction were identified at sites with and without laboratory computers among nurses in different types of nursing units (critical care or general care), or by age of the respondent. The response at different-sized hospitals could not be examined since all large and medium-sized hospitals in the study had laboratory computers.

Satisfaction levels of approximately 875 providers in the outpatient clinics of hospitals with laboratory computers were compared with satisfaction levels of approximately 425 clinic providers in hospitals with no laboratory system. The effects of the laboratory computer on the laboratory ordering and laboratory results factors were examined.

Results of the analyses are shown in Table 3-2. In outpatient settings, the only significant difference associated with the computers was that the presence of a laboratory computer was associated with *lower* satisfaction with laboratory results for outpatients. Satisfaction with laboratory results for outpatients at sites with laboratory computers was 2.86 and at sites without laboratory computers, satisfaction was 3.32. Although it initially appeared that having a laboratory computer affected satisfaction with laboratory ordering, when size was entered into the analysis as a covariate, the differences in satisfaction with

Table 3-2. Comparison of Satisfaction Levels at Sites With and Without Departmental Computer Systems (Mean Likert Values)

Satisfaction Factors	No Lab Computer	Lab Computer	Difference (Computer-No Computer)
Laboratory results (nurses)	2.71	2.98	+0.27
Laboratory turnaround (nurses)	2.70	2.72	N.S.S.[1]
Laboratory results for outpatients (physicians)	3.32	2.86	-0.46
Laboratory ordering for outpatients (physicians)	3.47	3.26	_[2]
Laboratory results for inpatients (physicians)	2.47	2.02	-0.45
	No Pharmacy Computer	**Pharmacy Computer**	**Difference (Computer-No Computer)**
Medication information (nurses)	3.72	3.63	_[2]
Medication information for outpatients (physicians)	2.55	2.61	+0.06
Medication information for inpatients (physicians)	2.44	2.31	-0.13

[1]Difference not statistically significant.
[2]More detailed analysis (two-way ANOVA) revealed this effect could be explained by differences in facility size.

laboratory ordering for outpatients was found to be explained by facility size alone.

The comparison of satisfaction of 735 inpatient care physicians at sites with laboratory computers and 340 physicians at sites without laboratory computers revealed a *lower* level of satisfaction with laboratory information at sites with laboratory computers. As shown in Table 3-2, satisfaction with laboratory results for inpatients was 2.02 at sites with laboratory computers and 2.47 at sites without laboratory computers.

A statistically significant difference in satisfaction was found at sites with and without computers among different specialty groups for the laboratory results factor. However, there was no consistent pattern to these responses. There were no statistically significant differences in the response to laboratory computers between providers in primary care and specialty clinics, or among providers of different ages, and no consistent trend in satisfaction differences according to the size of the facility.

Information Satisfaction Associated with Pharmacy Computers

Satisfaction levels of approximately 865 nurses in 10 hospitals with pharmacy systems were compared with responses from approximately 255 nurses in four hospitals without pharmacy systems. One factor was examined: medication information. Results are summarized in Table 3-2. The initial analysis indicated that nurses at hospitals with pharmacy computers had lower levels of satisfaction with the medication information than nurses in hospitals without pharmacy systems. However, when size was included as a covariate, the overall difference in satisfaction with medication information was found to be related to differences in satisfaction at hospitals of different sizes.

To examine the effects of a pharmacy system on outpatient medication information, the satisfaction of 1,040 providers in the clinics with pharmacy department computers was compared with satisfaction levels of approximately 260 providers in four clinics without pharmacy department computers. Having a pharmacy computer was associated with a slightly higher satisfaction with the outpatient medication information factor. No consistent trend emerged in satisfaction with outpatient information medication according to size of facility and there were no statistically significant differences between providers in primary care and specialty clinics, or among providers of different ages.

The satisfaction of 210 physicians who provided inpatient care at sites without pharmacy computers was compared with satisfaction levels of 850 physicians at sites with pharmacy computers. Physicians at sites with pharmacy systems had slightly *lower* levels of satisfaction than those with medication information.

There were statistically significant differences in satisfaction at sites with and without computers among different specialty groups for the factor related to medication information. However, there was no consistent pattern to these responses that would support a conclusion that one specialty received more benefit from departmental automation than another.

Conclusions about Satisfaction Associated with Pharmacy and Laboratory Department Computers

The study of departmental systems showed little association between having a departmental computer and nurses' and physicians' satisfaction with related information.

The only significant association between having a laboratory computer and nurses' satisfaction was for the laboratory results process factor. Satisfaction with this factor was 0.27 higher (on a five-point scale) among nurses at hospitals with laboratory department computers. This improvement was probably related to the fact that with a departmental laboratory computer, results are less likely to be lost than with manual information processes. In the four hospitals where terminals were available in patient care areas, the nurse could quickly retrieve laboratory results on a computer terminal in the patient care areas. At other sites, the nurses could call the laboratory and ask for a result to be looked up on a terminal in the laboratory.

The lack of correlation between having a departmental computer and higher nursing satisfaction with the factors related to turnaround time for laboratory results and medication information may be related to the fact that the departmental automation did not support complete processes from the nursing perspective. With a departmental laboratory system, the order still had to be manually transmitted to the laboratory; this part of total turnaround time was not affected. Nurses had no direct access to information in the pharmacy system. It is not unreasonable to conclude that nurses found it frustrating that critical clinical information was readily available within the pharmacy but not accessible to nurses who were providing direct patient care.

The analysis of the relationship between providers' satisfaction with outpatient information and the presence of clinical computers within the laboratory and pharmacy revealed a limited number of statistically significant differences associated with having a departmental computer. The largest difference was that satisfaction with laboratory information was *lower* at sites with laboratory computers than at sites without laboratory computers. For outpatient information, the contrast was a value of 2.86 at sites with a computer versus 3.32 at sites without a laboratory computer, and for inpatient information the difference was 2.02 at sites with laboratory computers versus 2.47 at sites without computers. The negative association between physician satisfaction and having a laboratory computer was unexpected. Since two thirds of the test sites had computer terminals in a central location within high-volume outpatient clinics and inpatient units for use in looking up test results, it was expected that the physicians' satisfaction with laboratory results information would improve. It may be that by making information available, but not providing convenient access to that information (e.g., no access in the outpatient exam rooms, physicians' office, or inpatient bedside) raised expectations and decreased satisfaction.

Although having a pharmacy system was associated with a statistically significant, positive difference in physicians' satisfaction with medication information for outpatients, the magnitude of the difference (+0.06 on a 5.0 scale) would probably not be seen as an incentive to buy pharmacy computers. Having a pharmacy system was associated with a significant, but also small, negative difference (-0.11) in satisfaction for questions related to medication information for inpatients.

The small positive and many negative differences associated with departmental computers led us to an overall conclusion that computers installed in clinical departments have very little positive effect on nurses' and physicians' satisfaction with clinical information. Despite the fact that 57 percent of U.S. hospitals have acquired departmental computers in their pharmacies, and 43 percent have acquired such systems for their laboratories(1), our research indicates these investments probably provide little direct benefit in increasing the satisfaction of the key users of this information–nurses and physicians.

Physicians' and Nurses' Satisfaction with an Integrated Patient Care System

A second case study involved examining changes in satisfaction when the CHCS system was installed in five of the hospitals where baseline satisfaction was measured. Changes in satisfaction were also measured in three control hospitals that did not receive the CHCS system. The hospitals included in the study of the CHCS included the smallest and largest hospitals in the baseline study plus three midsized hospitals. The CHCS system was still under development at the time of this study and the capabilities designed to support nursing care processes (patient assessment, care planning, and charting) had not yet been implemented. Therefore, it was expected that the CHCS system would have had little impact on nurses' satisfaction with information and the study of changes in nurses' satisfaction was conducted only at three CHCS and the three control sites. (As will be discussed later, this assumption about changes in nurses' satisfaction was disproven by the results of the study.)

Clearly, the information needs for inpatient and outpatient care are different. In inpatient care, a high volume of information must be obtained and managed for a short period of time. In outpatient care, the volume of information is less, but information obtained at one visit may be used months or years later. In inpatient care, clerical staff, nurses, house officers and staff physicians assume different roles in information management. In outpatient care, the physician treating the patient has little support in compiling information, transcribing orders, and tracking down lost or missing information. When inpatient care is delivered, the medical record is retained on the patient floor. The outpatient record may be transferred among many clinics as the patient obtains care; therefore, the record may be unavailable when needed to review information or record the results of tests and treatment. Because of the differences in information needs and manual processes, the impact of computers may be different in inpatient and outpatient settings. We could find no prior studies that examined this hypothesis.

Some early research indicated that there may be differences in acceptance of patient care information systems between physicians and nurses; however, a computer-based patient record system must be acceptable to both. Because we examined the impact of the same patient care information system on the satisfaction of physicians who practiced in both inpatient and outpatient settings, and of nurses and physicians in the same inpatient settings, we used the data to determine whether the integrated clinical computer system being evaluated was acceptable to both physicians and nurses who provide inpatient care, and to determine if the system effectively supported physicians in providing both inpatient and outpatient care. Therefore, the findings of this case study were analyzed to answer two questions:

- Does the availability of an integrated patient care information system have similar impacts on physicians' satisfaction with information to support inpatient and outpatient care?
- Does the availability of an integrated patient care information system have similar impacts on physicians' and nurses' satisfaction with information to support inpatient care?

In addition to providing detailed comparative data, this case study differs from most past research in that survey data were obtained from several different hospitals, whereas most past research focused on one or two sites. Community as well as teaching hospitals were included, whereas most prior research has been conducted in teaching hospitals.

The capabilities of the CHCS system were described in the introduction to this chapter. We monitored the installation of the CHCS and, before the postimplementation satisfaction surveys were distributed, the status of system implementation was reviewed to ensure that the CHCS computer system was being used routinely in patient care delivery. All the sites included in the case study met these criteria.

Introduction to the Design of the CHCS Case Study

Satisfaction with information following CHCS installation was collected using a paper survey. The survey included the information-related and general satisfaction questions that were described in the earlier case study. Sixteen of the inpatient information items were included on both the physician and nursing surveys; these items were used to compare changes in physicians' and nurses' satisfaction. Sixteen information items on the physician survey were asked in both inpatient and outpatient settings; these were used to compare changes in physicians' satisfaction with inpatient and outpatient information.

The survey fielded after the CHCS system was installed contained additional questions related to use of the CHCS system and benefits received. Physicians and nurses were asked about their level of agreement with a series of positively and negatively worded statements about use of the system (e.g., how easy it was to use, usefulness of screen layouts, access to computer terminals, impact on efficiency). Responses were recorded on a five-point scale: strongly agree (5), agree somewhat (4), neutral (3), disagree somewhat (2), and strongly disagree (1). The post-implementation survey also contained questions about the level and type of use of the system by each respondent.

As in the baseline case study, all physicians and nurses who provided direct patient care received the survey. All inpatient nurses and all physicians at three sites were included in the survey. At two sites, a random sample of 50 percent of the physicians received the CHCS satisfaction survey. (The remaining physicians received a different survey for another study.) Surveys were distributed and returned through the hospital mail system. Since staffing records did not distinguish between physicians who provide outpatient care, or care in both settings, instructions on the survey directed the respondent to complete only those sections that related to the setting(s) in which they currently practiced. The physician contrasts described in this paper include only providers who answered both sets of questions. (Eighty percent of physicians in the baseline survey and 61 percent of the respondents in the CHCS survey provided both inpatient and outpatient care.)

The overall response rate to the physician survey at the five sites was 60 percent in the baseline and 79 percent in the CHCS study period. For nurses at the three study sites, response rates were 86 percent in the baseline and 65 percent in the CHCS study period.

Responses to individual questions were grouped together into factors to facilitate the analysis. More factors were created for this case study since the CHCS system was expected to affect many different information processes. Since we could only use questions that were available for both groups being compared, we created two sets of factors: one to contrast changes in nurses' and physicians' satisfaction with information support for inpatient care, and the other to contrast changes in physicians' satisfaction with information for inpatient and outpatient care. The factors used to compare physicians' satisfaction with inpatient and outpatient information are shown in Table 3-3 and the factors used in the comparison of physicians' and nurses' satisfaction with inpatient information are shown in Table 3-4. The tables display the survey questions that made up each factor. Effective reliability of the factors (calculated using the Spearman-Brown formula) ranged from 0.57 to 0.92.

Table 3-3. Factors Used to Compare Physician Satisfaction with Outpatient and Inpatient Information

Laboratory Information

- Ease of ordering laboratory tests
- Turnaround time for STAT laboratory test results
- Turnaround time for routine laboratory test results
- The process for notifying you about abnormal laboratory test results

Radiology Information

- Turnaround time for STAT radiology reports
- The process for notifying you about abnormal radiology reports
- Ease of ordering radiology procedures

Medication Information

- Availability of information on medication allergies
- Completeness of outpatient medication profiles/inpatient medication administration record

Availability and Quality of Records

- Availability of outpatient record at time of visit/ability to find the current inpatient record when you need it

Availability and Quality of Records (continued)

- Availability of outpatient records for telephone consults/availability of inpatient records from prior admissions
- Legibility of elements in records
- Time it takes to locate information in records

Ordering

- Ease of ordering laboratory tests
- Ease of ordering radiology procedures

Retrieving Results

- Turnaround time for STAT laboratory test results
- Turnaround time for routine laboratory test results
- The process for notifying you about abnormal laboratory test results
- Turnaround time for STAT radiology reports
- The process for notifying you about abnormal radiology reports

Time Locating Information

- Time you spend locating test results
- Time it takes to locate information in patient records

Table 3-4. Factors Used to Compare Physician and Nurse Satisfaction with Inpatient Information

Laboratory Information

- The process for notifying providers about abnormal laboratory diagnostic results
- Time you spend locating laboratory test results
- Ease of ordering laboratory tests
- Accuracy of test results in inpatient records
- Turnabout time for return of STAT laboratory test results
- Turnaround time for return of routine laboratory test results

Radiology Information

- Ease of ordering radiology procedures
- Turnaround time for return of STAT radiology reports
- The process for notifying providers about abnormal radiology reports
- Time you spend locating radiology reports

Medication Records

- Completeness of information on patient's medication record
- Accuracy of medication administration record in inpatient record

Availability and Quality of Records

- Ability to find the current inpatient record when you need it
- Availability of inpatient records from prior admissions
- Legibility of elements in the inpatient record
- Time it takes to locate information in the patient chart

Ordering

- Ease of ordering laboratory tests
- Ease of ordering radiology procedures

Retrieving Results

- Turnaround time for return of STAT laboratory test results
- Turnaround time for return of routine laboratory test results
- Turnaround time for return of STAT radiology reports
- The process for notifying providers about abnormal radiology reports
- The process for notifying providers about abnormal laboratory test results

Time Locating Information

- Time you spend locating laboratory test results
- Time you spend locating radiology reports
- Time it takes to locate information in the patient chart
- Amount of paperwork

Physicians' and nurses' responses to the CHCS in inpatient care were compared using two-way ANOVA with automation (baseline or CHCS) and type of staff (nurse or physician) as the two independent variables. The analysis was designed to examine differences in the changes in satisfaction among nurses and among physicians.

The analysis comparing physicians' and nurses' responses was performed with and without the one general question, "Overall how satisfied are you with your practice at name of hospital," as a covariate to adjust for other changes between the two periods that might have affected nurses and physicians differently. While the presence of the overall question as a covariate did explain more of the total variation in satisfaction, it did not alter the conclusions about differences in response to the CHCS. The results presented here are not adjusted for the response to the general satisfaction question.

Physicians' reactions to computer support in inpatient and outpatient care were also compared using two-way ANOVA with automation (baseline versus CHCS) and setting (inpatient versus outpatient) as the independent variables. This analysis took advantage of the fact that the same respondents answered questions about inpatient and outpatient information. Therefore, it was not necessary to adjust for individual differences in general satisfaction levels.

As mentioned in the introduction to this case study, baseline and post-CHCS satisfaction information was also collected at three control sites that had no change in automation. As a first step in the analysis, satisfaction changes in test sites were compared with satisfaction changes at the control sites. The purpose of this contrast was to determine if changes other than the CHCS had affected satisfaction with information.

The baseline satisfaction levels at test and control sites and the changes that occurred from the baseline to the CHCS time period are shown in Table 3-5. Baseline satisfaction at control sites was either the same as or slightly higher than baseline satisfaction at sites that received the CHCS system. Overall general (noninformation) satisfaction increased at both test and control sites. The differences in these changes were not statistically significant. For nurses, there were small changes in satisfaction with information at control sites and major changes at test sites. This increased our confidence that the changes observed were attributable to the CHCS system.

When changes in physicians' satisfaction with outpatient information at test sites were compared with changes at control sites, the positive changes at test sites were significant for all factors except radiology results. This led us to conclude that changes in other areas could be attributed to the CHCS system.

There were no significant differences in changes in physicians' satisfaction with inpatient information at test and control sites. This led us to conclude that installation of the CHCS system did not result in a measurable change in physicians' satisfaction with inpatient information.

Table 3-5. Comparison of Changes in Satisfaction at CHCS (Test) and Control Sites (Mean Likert Values)

Nurses' Satisfaction	Baseline at Test Sites	Baseline at Control Sites	Changes at CHCS (Test Sites)	Changes at Control Sites
Overall satisfaction with information	2.96	3.10	+0.44	-0.02
• Lab results	2.74	3.04	+0.76	-0.14
• Radiology results	3.06	3.23	+0.42	-0.04
• Medication administration	3.78	3.77	-0.79	-0.05
Overall general satisfaction	3.04	3.06	+0.44	+0.37*
Physicians' Satisfaction				
Overall satisfaction with outpatient information	2.79	2.81	+0.69	+0.10
• Outpatient laboratory results	3.14	3.34	+0.49	-0.33
• Outpatient radiology results	3.28	3.14	+0.21	+0.15*
• Outpatient medication information	2.55	2.71	+1.18	+0.16
Overall satisfaction with inpatient information	3.11	3.12	0.0	+0.09*
• Inpatient laboratory results	3.18	3.35	+0.13	-0.10*
• Inpatient radiology results	3.29	3.17	-0.13	+0.14*
Overall general satisfaction	3.16	3.25	+0.32	+0.36*

*Difference in change at test and control sites not statistically significant.

Results

Contrasts in Physicians' and Nurses' Satisfaction Response
to an Integrated Patient Care Computer System in Inpatient Care

Nurses and physicians had similar levels of experience with the CHCS. Fifty-eight percent of physicians and 49 percent of nurses reported that they had used the system for more than 1 year, and 19 percent of physicians and 18 percent of nurses had used the system for more than 1 but less than 6 months.

The effect of the CHCS on physicians' and nurses' satisfaction with inpatient information was compared for seven factors: laboratory information, radiology information, pharmacy information, the availability and quality of the medical record, the process for ordering tests, the process for retrieving results, and time spent in information handling. Results are shown in Table 3-6. All satisfaction levels are average responses for all questions in the factor.

For six of the seven information factors related to inpatient care, changes in nurses' satisfaction were significantly more positive than changes in physicians' satisfaction. The improvement in satisfaction with time spent in information handling was significantly higher for nurses (+0.83) than for physicians (+0.21), and the improvement in satisfaction with laboratory information among nurses (+0.88) was significantly higher than the satisfaction improvement among physicians (+0.03). For four factors (radiology information, record access and quality, ordering, and results reporting) nurses' satisfaction improved after the CHCS was installed and physicians' satisfaction declined. The biggest difference in response for these factors was with ordering tests, where physicians' satisfaction declined by -0.77 scale points while nurses' satisfaction increased by +0.52 scale points. The difference between the drop in satisfaction with medication information for physicians (-0.59) and nurses (-0.78) was not statistically significant.

Physicians' and nurses' opinions about use of the CHCS system are shown on Table 3-7. All responses are on a five-point scale from strongly agree (5) to strongly disagree (1). (The mean response to these questions was compared using a Wilcoxon two-sample test.) Physicians and nurses agreed that CHCS terminals were available when needed. For other aspects of CHCS use, nurses rated the system significantly more positively than physicians. The largest difference in response was for the item related to the impact of CHCS on individual productivity.

Respondents were also asked how frequently they used the system for entering medication or other orders, retrieving results, and for electronic mail. Responses were recorded on a scale ranging from many times a day to never. Reported levels of usage among physicians and nurses are shown in Table 3-8. A higher percentage of physicians reported using the system many times per day to enter information, whereas a higher percentage of nurses reported using the system frequently for retrieving results for inpatients.

Table 3-6. Comparison of Physicians' and Nurses' Satisfaction with CHCS Support for Inpatient Information (Mean Likert Values)

Information Factor	Physicians			Nurses		
	Satisfaction Level in Baseline	Satisfaction Level with CHCS	Change in Satisfaction	Satisfaction Level in Baseline	Satisfaction Level with CHCS	Change in Satisfaction
Time in information handling	2.33	2.54	+0.21	2.40	3.23	+0.83
Laboratory Information	3.10	3.13	0.03	2.70	3.58	+0.88
Radiology information	2.98	2.77	-0.21	2.91	3.31	+0.40
Record access and quality	3.37	3.09	-0.28	3.30	3.66	+0.36
Ordering	3.59	2.82	-0.77	3.15	3.67	+0.52
Results reporting	3.07	2.94	-0.13	2.70	3.21	+0.51
Medication information	3.51	2.92	-0.59[1]	3.78	3.00	+-0.78[1]

[1]Difference in response between nurses and physicians is not statistically significant.

Table 3-7. Comparison of Physicians' and Nurses' Opinions about the CHCS (Mean Likert Values)

Survey Item	Level of Agreement by Physicians	Level of Agreement by Nurses
CHCS terminals are available where needed	3.8[1]	4.0[1]
Received good training in the use of CHCS	3.3	3.7
CHCS *is not* easy to use	3.6	3.1
CHCS screens are designed to be easy to use	2.7	3.1
CHCS is incorporated easily into patient care	2.6	2.9
CHCS makes me *less* productive	3.5	2.6

[1]Difference in response between nurses and physicians is not statistically significant.

Table 3-8. Use of the CHCS by Physicians and Nurses

Frequency of Use	Type of Use (% of Respondents)							
	Entering Medications/Other Information		Retrieving Results--Inpatients		Electronic Mail		Retrieving Results--Outpatients	
	MDs	RNs	MDs	RNs	MDs	RNs	MDs	RNs
Many times per day	79	31	33	51	50	42	69	NA
At least once per day	11	25	20	30	35	49	18	NA
Two-three times per week	5	11	16	11	9	5	9	NA
Once per week	3	8	16	5	4	4	3	NA
Rarely/never	2	24	15	2	2	0	1	NA

Contrasts in Physicians' Response to an Integrated Patient Care Computer System in Inpatient versus Outpatient Care

The satisfaction levels of approximately 180 physicians who provided inpatient and outpatient care using the CHCS were compared with 280 physicians who provided inpatient and outpatient care before the CHCS system was installed. The analysis was designed to examine changes in satisfaction in inpatient versus outpatient care settings that occurred between the baseline period and after the CHCS was in use.

Summary results for seven information factors are shown in Table 3-9. The differences in physicians' responses to the CHCS in inpatient and outpatient care were all statistically significant. There was a consistently more positive response to CHCS in the outpatient setting. Satisfaction with radiology information decreased in both settings; however, the decrease was significantly greater for inpatient care (-0.33) than for outpatient care (-0.17). Satisfaction with time spent locating information increased in both settings; however, the increase was significantly greater in outpatient care (+1.15) than inpatient care (+0.32).

Satisfaction with five other factors (laboratory information, medication information, record access and quality, ordering, and retrieving results) increased after the CHCS support was available in the outpatient setting and decreased for the inpatient setting. The largest differences in response to the computer were for the factors related to record access and quality (+1.00 for outpatient care and -0.13 for inpatient care) and for medication information (+0.88 for outpatient care and –0.14 for inpatient care).

The use of the system by physicians in inpatient and outpatient care differed. The major difference was in the process for ordering tests and medications. In outpatient care, physicians entered all orders. For inpatient care, only one site (a major teaching hospital) required physicians to use the system for entering orders. At one site all inpatient ordering was performed by pharmacy staff (medication orders) and nursing (all other orders). At the remaining sites, inpatient medication orders were entered by the pharmacy staff; other inpatient orders were entered by a mix of staff from ancillary clinical departments, nursing, and physician staff.

While no statistical tests were performed, inspection of the data from individual sites indicated that physicians' satisfaction with completeness of medication records and ease of ordering tests and procedures declined independent of the method used for entering orders (see Table 3-10). In fact, the magnitude of the decline in satisfaction was lowest at the site where all inpatient orders were entered by the physicians.

Table 3-9. Comparison of Physicians' Satisfaction with CHCS Support for Inpatient and Outpatient Information (Mean Likert Values)

Information Factor	Inpatient			Outpatient		
	Satisfaction Level in Baseline	Satisfaction Level with CHCS	Change in Satisfaction	Satisfaction Level in Baseline	Satisfaction Level with CHCS	Change in Satisfaction
Time locating information	2.67	2.99	+0.32	2.18	3.33	+1.15
Laboratory Information	3.24	3.15	-0.09	2.99	3.21	+0.22
Radiology information	3.22	2.89	-0.33	3.07	2.90	-0.17
Medication information	3.40	3.26	-0.14	2.68	3.50	+0.88
Record access and quality	3.34	3.21	-0.13	2.71	3.71	+1.00
Ordering	3.59	3.10	-0.49	3.23	3.29	+0.06
Retrieving results	3.08	3.01	-0.07	2.93	3.01	+0.08

Table 3-10. Comparison of Three Approaches for Entering Inpatient Orders (Mean Likert Values)

Method of Order Entry for Inpatients		Satisfaction with Completeness of Medication Records	Satisfaction with Ease of Ordering Radiology Tests	Satisfaction with Ease of Ordering Laboratory Tests
All inpatient orders by MD; RN charting of inpatient medications	Baseline	3.38	3.26	3.71
	CHCS	3.09	3.17	3.27
	Change	-0.29	-0.09	-0.44
All inpatient medication orders by pharmacy; all remaining inpatient orders by nursing; no charting	Baseline	3.64	3.28	3.75
	CHCS	3.04	3.00	3.07
	Change	-0.60	-0.28	-0.68
All inpatient medication orders by pharmacy; remaining orders by MD, RN, or ancillary; no charting	Baseline	3.39	3.61	3.81
	CHCS	3.07	3.19	3.05
	Change	-0.32	-0.42	-0.76

Conclusions about Satisfaction with a Patient Care Information System

After the CHCS system was installed, the largest gains in satisfaction were among outpatient physicians, followed by inpatient nurses, and then inpatient physicians.

Comparisons of Physicians and Nurses

Both physicians and nurses reported that they were frequent users of the CHCS. Ninety percent of physicians reported using the system at least once per day for entering information–most reported using this function many times per day. Since physicians were required to use the system to enter outpatient orders, this result is not surprising. Use of the system to retrieve results was voluntary because traditional paper charts were still maintained. Fifty-one percent of the nurses and 33 percent of the physicians reported that they used the CHCS many times a day to retrieve inpatient results, and 69 percent of the physicians reported using the system many times per day to retrieve results for outpatients. Over 80 percent of both physicians and nurses used the system at least daily for electronic mail.

A 1985 study indicated that at Boston's Beth Israel Hospital, 80 percent of physicians and nurses who had used their computer system at least 10 times indicated they used the system "most of the time" to retrieve results.(5) The Beth Israel system had been in routine use since 1980. It supported access to clinical results, registration information, and medical databases, but was not used by physicians or nurses for entering orders. These data are not directly comparable to the results of the CHCS study; however, they both support a conclusion that both of these patient care information systems were routinely used by many physicians and nurses.

After the CHCS was installed, physicians and nurses were less satisfied with the factor related to inpatient medication information. This factor contained two items: completeness of information on the patient's medication administration record and accuracy of the information on the medication record. With the CHCS, inpatient medication orders were entered into the system, but at the three sites where physicians' and nurses' satisfaction levels were compared, the CHCS was not used to record information on medication administration. The decline in satisfaction with medication records may be due to rising expectations. The physicians and nurses may have felt that the level of automated support they received with the CHCS was unacceptable compared with their expectations. However, it may also be true that the use of the CHCS system increased errors or created gaps in medication records.

Both physicians and nurses reported that after the CHCS was installed, they were more satisfied with the time spent in retrieving test results and in finding patient information. Since the CHCS operated in parallel with a traditional paper chart, and gave them another, optional source of information, this finding is not surprising.

It is more difficult to explain the fact that for the inpatient information factors related to radiology information record access and quality, ordering, and results reporting, nurses' satisfaction *increased* and physicians' satisfaction declined. It was expected that nurses' satisfaction would be unaffected by the current functions of the CHCS, because traditional "nursing" applications of assessment, care planning, and charting were not supported. Conversely, it was expected that improved access to clinical data would be a real benefit for physicians.

One explanation for the greater change in satisfaction with inpatient information among nurses using the CHCS is that the nurses' role in managing inpatient information was underestimated. Another explanation is that physicians' use of the CHCS may have produced corollary benefits for nurses. At most CHCS sites, nurses no longer needed to transcribe all physicians' orders from order sheets to the proper forms since physicians or pharmacists took over responsibility for entering at least some of the orders directly into the CHCS. In informal interviews, nurses also reported that they spent less time trying to locate test results for the physicians, since physicians used the CHCS system to look up information on test status or results.

The comparison of opinions about the CHCS indicates a third explanation for the difference in response between physicians and nurses. Physicians were more likely to agree with the statement that the CHCS was not easy to use. Physicians also agreed that the CHCS made them less productive, while nurses disagreed with this statement. It may be that the system design was better suited for typical nursing uses such as looking up a result for a patient than for physicians who wanted to evaluate trends in many results over time or needed access to different types of information.

A recent study of the sources of information to answer questions posed at physicians' clinical rounds indicates that only about one half of the questions could be answered with information in the medical record alone.(6) The remaining questions required access to textbooks, the medical literature, or medical databases. Because the CHCS did not support access to outside databases or literature, it may have solved fewer of the physicians' problems with access to information.

The findings of this study are similar to satisfaction survey results from a study conducted nearly two decades ago of the Technicon system at El Camino Hospital. Nurses were more positive about system benefits than physicians. Nurses were at least twice as likely to agree that the computer system increased the efficiency of their work, improved quality of care, and contributed to better functioning of the hospital. Physicians were more than twice as likely to concur that the new computer system was no better than the old way and that the system did not perform as they expected. The authors did not speculate on why this difference occurred.(7) With both the Technicon and CHCS systems, physicians had to assume a greater role in order and results management. This change in responsibility may have been responsible for the observed differences in satisfaction.

In the Bleich study cited earlier(5), physicians and nurses were asked about the helpfulness of the computer. Eighty-nine percent of the respondents reported the computer was *very helpful*. Although details are not given, the authors state that ratings were similar for staff physicians, nurses, and house officers. However, this system was used most frequently by physicians and nurses for the same function–to retrieve test results–and all use of the system was voluntary.

A comparison of physicians' and nurses' satisfaction with an ICU data management system conducted in 1990 indicated that while overall satisfaction was the same for physicians and nurses, physicians were less positive about the display format, and nurses were more satisfied with the data entry aspects of the system. Physicians were less convinced that the computer improved access to information. The authors concluded that the system needed to be redesigned to support physicians.(8)

Although studies identified in the literature are not directly comparable to the findings of our research, they do help to illustrate some of the factors that may influence satisfaction with a computer system. Since physicians and nurses use systems for different types of tasks, a design may work well for one group of users and not another. Also, the functions supported by the computer may provide complete patient care information for one group, but not the other. It is likely that similar differences would be found with respiratory therapists, social workers, and other groups that provide patient care. This indicates that nurses and physicians need different "views" of patient data. As discussed in Chapter 4, future developers and purchasers of information systems should ensure that this flexibility is built into any patient care computer system.

Comparisons of Inpatient and Outpatient Care

Physicians were less satisfied with CHCS benefits to inpatient care than outpatient care. Satisfaction with laboratory information, medication information, record access and quality, ease of ordering, and retrieving results all declined after the system was used to support inpatient care, but increased when the system was used to support outpatient care. The three areas with the greatest increase in outpatient satisfaction (medication information, record access and quality, and time locating information) were all rated as unsatisfactory (below 3) in the baseline.

One explanation for the increases in outpatient satisfaction is that there are more problems managing outpatient information in a manual system. Outpatient records are more apt to be lost and they are less likely to be kept in a standard format. Also, because of the long time delays between visits, information that is missing at the time of an outpatient visit is very difficult to locate, and there are typically few supporting staff to help locate old records and old information. By providing a reliable source of information to substitute for or augment the paper chart, the CHCS may have produced more changes in access to information in outpatient care settings. This explanation is consistent with the fact that some of the largest increases in satisfaction were associated with outpatient factors where baseline satisfaction was rated as unsatisfactory.

However, differences in the baseline availability and quality of inpatient and outpatient information do not account for the consistent decline in satisfaction with inpatient information, nor does this explain the fact that for some factors, satisfaction levels were higher in outpatient care than in inpatient care after the CHCS was installed. It appears that the CHCS had benefits that made system use valuable for physicians in the outpatient care area but not for inpatient care.

The comparison of the impact of the CHCS on satisfaction with ordering refutes conventional wisdom. It was expected that physicians would be dissatisfied with a system that required them to enter orders. However, satisfaction with ordering did not decline in outpatient care when physicians were required to use the CHCS for ordering. Physicians' satisfaction with ordering declined in inpatient care irrespective of whether or not physicians were required to enter orders.

Cautions in Interpreting Case Study Results

Although this evaluation provided a comprehensive analysis of nurses' and physicians' satisfaction with a patient care information system, there are many other important measures of the effect of the system that also need to be studied (e.g., quality of care, access to care, and cost). This case study does not provide the data necessary to reach conclusions about the overall value of the CHCS in supporting patient care delivery.

Only one of the wide variety of currently available patient care information systems was included in this case study. Other systems differ in the capabilities they include, in the way they present information to users, and the method required for entering information. Because no directly comparable satisfaction data from evaluations of other health care information systems were found in the literature, it is not possible to determine how well the study findings represent the state of the art of patient care information systems.

Implications

Many organizations are lobbying for increased use of computer-based records. The Institute of Medicine has called for a national initiative to convert to computer-based patient records.(9) The Joint Commission on Accreditation of Health Care Organizations has added information management to its standards for accreditation(10), and there is a continual flow of national initiatives to increase the availability of health care data. The results of this second case study indicate that there may be differences in the automation needs and priorities of nurses and physicians, and in inpatient and outpatient care settings. A computer-based patient record should satisfy all the requirements for these different users and work environments.

Our findings reinforce the need to fund demonstration projects to gain additional information about the benefits and acceptance of computer systems in patient care delivery. These demonstration projects should be conducted in inpatient and outpatient settings and solicit information from physicians and nurses. Results of this case study indicate that particular attention should be paid to understanding the causes of dissatisfaction with computer support for inpatient information among physicians, support for medication records in inpatient care, and support of radiology reporting. Carefully controlled studies that include comparisons of the same settings before and after automation will be needed to isolate the effects of the pilot computer systems from the many other variables affecting patient care outcomes, costs, and physicians' and nurses' satisfaction.

References

1. Dorenfest SI. Hospital Information Systems: the State of the Art. Chicago: Sheldon Dorenfest Associates Limited, 1992.
2. Andrews W. '92 Bedside systems report. Healthcare Informatics 1992;9:56-61.
3. Drazen EL. Physicians' and Nurses' Satisfaction with Clinical Computer Systems, A thesis submitted to the faculty of the Harvard School of Public Health, Boston, MA, 1992.
4. AHA Hospital Statistics, Chicago, IL, AHA publishers:1991.
5. Bleich HL, Beckley RF, Howowitz GL, et al. Clinical computing in a teaching hospital. New England Journal of Medicine 1985;312:756-764.
6. Osheroff JA, Forsythe DE, Buchanan BG, Bankowitz RA, Blumfeld BH, Miller RA. Physicians' information needs: analysis of questions posed during clinical teaching.Annals of Internal Medicine 1991;114:576-581.
7. Battelle Memorial Institute. Evaluation of the Implementation of a Medical Information System at a General Community Hospital. Arlington, VA:NTIS 1973.
8. Gilhoolly KJ, Logie R, Ross D, Ramayya P, Green C. Users' perceptions of a computerized information system in intensive care (ABICUS) on introduction and after two months of Use. International Journal of Clinical Monitoring and Computing 1991;8:101-106.
9. Dick RS, Steen EB. The Computer-Based Patient Record: An Essential Technology for Health Care. Washington, DC:National Academy Press, 1991.

10. JCAHO. Joint Standards for Information Management in Health Care Organizations (undated).

4
Designing Acceptable Patient Care Information Systems

Jane B. Metzger and Jonathan M. Teich

The state of the art of patient care information systems has been constantly advancing over the last 20 years. New database tools, faster computers, graphical interfaces, and automated instruments promise impressive benefits to patient care and practice management. To the physician or nurse evaluating a patient care information system, however, there is only one critical question, "Can I do my work more easily and effectively than I could before?" No system can bring about its promised benefits if it is not accepted and used.

An otherwise excellent system can fail to gain acceptance in many ways. If the system is unreliable, with slow response and long periods of downtime, it will be unacceptable. If users must spend long hours learning how to use it, they will receive it poorly. If the computer makes it hard for physicians or nurses to use patient information in a familiar pattern, or if entering and retrieving information is an awkward, time-consuming task, they are unlikely to perceive that the computer is a worthwhile investment.

No matter how many advances a patient care information system offers, it still represents a change in the way work is done in clinical practice. The effect of change is magnified as the system manages more patient information and physicians and nurses spend more and more of their time interacting with the system. A system that performs a discrete task such as look-up of laboratory results may be judged solely on a head-to-head comparison with the previous method; the effect of cultural change is small. If, on the other hand, the system is comprehensive, managing information for many aspects of practice, then the whole exceeds the sum of the parts. In this case, the system must not only provide superior data entry and retrieval tasks, but the entire process must serve the user as well or better than it did before.

We believe that the formula for success is simple: give physicians and nurses computer tools that offer substantial added value to their work, and make user interactions with the system as simple, efficient, and dependable as possible. Table 4-1 states the design and performance prerequisites that we believe are critical if a patient care information system is to be acceptable to physicians, nurses, and other providers. The order in which prerequisites are listed is not intended to convey any significance; in fact, successful systems should possess all of these attributes.

Using these criteria to organize the discussion, this chapter describes some of the principles of designing (or selecting) systems that are acceptable to physicians and nurses. This chapter draws from the published literature, from patient care information system evaluations and planning projects performed by Arthur D. Little over the last 20 years, and from the experience of clinical applications developers at the Brigham and Women's Hospital in Boston to explore these design prerequisites in detail.

Patient Care Information Systems Must Be Available Whenever Users Need Them to Manage Patient Care

Uptime and Downtime

Reliable system availability is a basic sine qua non for patient care information systems. Systems engineers tend to measure performance as "downtime" over some period of time. They further distinguish unplanned downtime from "planned" downtime, as needed for batch processing, backup, and recovery for many systems. For physicians and nurses, however, it matters not whether the period of unavailability is planned or not, or which component of the system is

Table 4-1. Design Prerequisites for Patient Care Information Systems

---

- Patient care information systems must be available whenever users need them to manage patient care.
- Patient care information systems must be available wherever decisions about care are made.
- Patient care information systems must provide quick and value-added access to information.
- Patient care information systems must be designed to fit actual patient care processes and work situations.
- Patient care information systems must be so easy to use that they require little (or no) training.
- Involving physicians with direct entry requires minimizing time and maximizing incentives.

---

the cause. These users need the system to be available any time they need to use patient information.

The implications of system reliability, and how these translate into technical requirements, depend upon the target patient care situation and the extent to which the patient care system has replaced traditional paper-based processes. Early clinical systems processed results for laboratory and radiology services so that physicians and nurses could consult a terminal at the nursing station instead of telephoning the laboratory. As a backup, daily results summaries were usually posted to patient charts and, when all else failed, users could resort to their old mode, the telephone, to obtain the information they needed. Planned downtime was usually scheduled at night, when few nurses or physicians were looking for patient data and few new diagnostic studies were being entered. In this clinical scenario, downtime was an inconvenience, especially if the system was unavailable when physicians needed to check on patient results, but it was not disruptive to patient care.

Once a system is processing orders, the stakes are higher. Since delays in communicating orders could result in delays in diagnosis or treatment, physicians, nurses, and other users demand a higher level of reliability. The consequences of downtime become more critical when physicians are entering orders directly, and are escalated further when nurses are relying upon system-generated due lists rather than transcribing orders onto a Kardex. In this situation, there is no paper trail from which to recreate the current care plan for each patient when the system crashes or has scheduled downtime. Understandably, both physicians and nurses become very intolerant of downtime and resist relying upon a system that is even occasionally unavailable when they need it.

In critical care areas such as an ICU, operating room, or Emergency Department, physicians and nurses capture and monitor many patient status indicators over time, and they typically order a large number of diagnostic studies. If they are to rely upon a patient care system to provide the flow sheets they use to track patient status and progress, they will expect "constant or very near constant availability" and will not accept a system that delivers less.(1)

When patient care information systems are supporting ambulatory care, system reliability increases in importance as the range of information available in the system database grows. Once the system replaces the paper medical record as the preferred information source, paper records are no longer routinely pulled. In this scenario, physicians may find it unacceptable to proceed with the clinic session when the system data upon which they rely are unavailable.

For advanced patient care information systems that approach a computer-based medical record, very high reliability standards are now stated. The Institute of Medicine study stated this requirement as "complete availability of the patient's record 24 hours a day for reading or updating–100 percent uptime."(2,3) This sets a performance target that is difficult for many current systems to achieve and may not be affordable. However, it is clear that increasing reliability–and providing backup and recovery in a way that is virtually invisible to users—must be a primary consideration in acquiring or expanding systems used in patient care.

Response Time

In addition to 24-hour availability, physician users expect the system to respond quickly to their input. Many own computers at home and use personal computers or microcomputer applications to manage business aspects of an office practice. They have come to expect a similar responsiveness in patient care information systems. Although the response time requirements of physician users have not been researched per se, research concerning computer user expectations in general has indicated that a 2-second response time (from the last keypress to the first usable information display) is appropriate for most routine tasks.(4) A 1- to 2-second response time is often cited for patient care information systems, even during peak periods of system usage, and physicians and other users of patient care information systems are sensitive to seconds or fractions of seconds of system delay.(5,6) Others have defined the acceptable response time as "think" time or "blink" time, in other words virtually imperceptible to the user.(2,7) (As systems in general use get faster, expectations regarding response time are moving in this direction.) However response time is expressed, physicians and other users of patient care information systems need response fast enough that they rarely feel they are waiting for the system.

Response time is particularly important for physicians because they tend to use a patient care system less constantly than many other users in health care. This means that they will probably sign on dozens of times each day and proceed to enter or retrieve patient information. Each of the multiple steps necessary to accomplish a task contributes to the total time that must be devoted, including log-on time.   In our experience, physicians in particular are more likely to complain about response time when they need to work through many screens (and wait for the system to process their input each time) to accomplish a simple task such as signing on to the system or identifying the patient of interest. Acceptable systems combine quick response time and a minimal number of user actions to accomplish each task.

Data Retention

Another measure of availability for patient care information systems is the capacity to provide access to patient history for as long as the information is likely to be clinically useful. This can take on a very different meaning for different patients and care scenarios; extensive online history is desirable in general, for legal as well as clinical reasons. It is important that policies and procedures for online retention, archiving, and purging of patient information be based on clinical considerations rather than dictated by system limitations. For example, laboratory results may be kept online for 1 year, but comprehensive summaries such as outpatient encounter histories and discharge abstracts should stay available much longer; allergies, if they are recorded on the computer, should be kept online for life. Even if first-tier storage is unavailable, systems should be able to archive data that are no longer needed and to retrieve needed information from archival storage in a reasonable period of time (i.e., in a few minutes).

Patient Care Information Systems Must Be Available Wherever Decisions About Care Are Made

Universal Access

If physicians and nurses are to use patient care information systems routinely, they must be able to access the system in all of the locations where they use patient information. This means that system terminals and printers should be located at nursing stations, offices, and other designated work areas throughout the hospital, the clinic, any off-site physician practice locations, and home. The farther away from the source, the more value is added to the access.

Ideally, in group work areas such as a nursing station or the Emergency Department, terminals are placed as close as possible to the work area and in sufficient numbers that physicians and nurses have immediate access. The system does not promote efficiency if users must walk many steps or wait to use a terminal.(5)

Needs on a specific unit depend upon the number of beds, the typical occupancy, patient acuity, and the extent of clinical support. On acute care units, a system that permits results retrieval may provide sufficient access with one terminal for every five to seven patients. Once nurses are charting nursing interventions (medication administration, vital signs, fluid intake/output) and physicians are using the system for order entry and results retrieval, this number may double. Fewer terminals may be needed on units where patients tend to have fewer orders and nursing interventions; more may be required on units that care for complex patients. Without renovations to work spaces and counters, it is often difficult to accommodate this number of terminals in close proximity to the chart rack, telephones, etc., where both nurses and physicians prefer to do their work.

Physicians we have interviewed who are doing both order entry and results retrieval for their inpatients often cite problems with access during busy times of the day such as morning rounds. This problem is particularly acute in a teaching hospital where numerous residents and staff physicians, and perhaps multiple teams of physicians, may be on the unit at the same time, and where physician rounds may also overlap with nursing shift change. In such cases, we have found that both nurses and physicians prefer to have some terminals designated for use by nurses and others designated for physician use. When there is insufficient space to accommodate all of these in the nursing station, some physician terminals can be located in a work area adjacent to the nursing station or in an office nearby.

Bedside Terminals

As patient care information systems have advanced over the last decade in particular, it has been suggested that physicians and nurses would derive more benefit if the computer was located at the site of the actual interaction with the patient. Initially, point-of-care access was designed for the acute medical/surgical care unit and brought fixed terminals to the patient room. Today, however, bedside terminals are used more widely in intensive care units. Specialized systems designed for intensive care assist the staff in managing, interpreting, and charting the data that flows from monitoring equipment and from numerous tests and procedures.(8)

Configurations for bedside terminals vary somewhat according to the basic layout and architecture of the nursing unit (open bays versus patient rooms, number of patient beds per room, etc.). In some settings bedside units are installed on metal arms to allow for bed movement and height adjustment.(9) Arthur D. Little surveys of nurse users in hospitals with bedside systems indicate that 80 percent believe this is the best location for a bedside terminal. (10) Ratios of terminals to patients vary with the scope of support, patient acuity, and unit layout, and can range from one terminal per patient in an intensive care unit to one per multipatient room or pod in an acute care unit.

The nursing functions most commonly performed on bedside terminals include charting of medications, vital signs, and fluid intake/output because this avoids redundant charting. Physical space limitations in patient rooms and the desirability of charting in the system away from patients and their visitors have, however, motivated some nurses to prefer charting at the nursing station.(11) Physicians have been shown to access patient data directly from the system more frequently when bedside units are available (9), but also want access outside patient rooms.

Physicians and nurses need access to system printers in patient care areas, as well as system terminals. At nursing stations, for example, results of diagnostic studies and consultations, nursing due lists and change-of-shift summaries, and rounds reports may be printed, depending upon the available features. Nurses prefer that printers for notifications and work documents such as due lists be at the nursing station where staff can periodically check for new output and keep an eye on paper supply, etc. When physicians are also requesting printed copies of products, such as rounds reports or patient lists, nurses prefer that an additional printer be dedicated to physician use, located in close proximity to physician work areas and terminals, so that both types of printing can occur simultaneously. Because of their superior print quality and quieter operation, laser printers are generally preferred over impact printers for hard copy.(12,13)

Outpatient Setting

In ambulatory care, point-of-care computing implies terminals in the offices of physicians and other providers. Physicians we have interviewed are not in favor of shared-use terminals in public areas such as hallways and break rooms because of the delay in gaining access (leaving the office and sometimes waiting in line) even if they only use the system to access diagnostic results. When the system includes physician-entered orders and reference information such as problem lists or notes, physicians express an even stronger need to access the system interactively during the encounter. They report that they will use the system differently if they have to leave their work area and the patient, not routinely consulting potentially valuable information such as each patient's medication history.

Depending upon how the clinic is arranged, a terminal in each office may suffice if at least some portion of each encounter (e.g., discussion and patient instructions at the conclusion) occurs in the office. Even if patients are never seen in the physician's office, a terminal is needed there to help in answering patient telephone queries, writing correspondence, and communicating with colleagues. However, in many clinics and practice settings almost all of the encounter occurs in an examination room, rather than in the physician's office. In this scenario, physicians find it extremely inconvenient to go to the office to access the system for information. Not surprisingly, in one installation of an ambulatory medical record system, physicians entered and updated patient problems, medications, and screening data more frequently when terminals were available in each examination room.(14)

Access in Other Areas

Inpatient units and clinics are the most obvious locations where care providers need access to a patient care system. However, many physicians and nurses are highly mobile during their work day. They may wish to review patient information in many additional locations, such as nonclinical areas, off-site practices, other hospitals, and their residence. Physicians and nurses can, therefore, benefit from computer access outside of patient care areas. In the hospital, terminals should be installed in lounges, medical libraries, dictation rooms, and resident work and call rooms to provide this access. If patient data are also to be used in teaching, terminals should be installed in conference rooms; for research access, terminals should also be placed in research offices/laboratories.

Many physicians who own and use computers in their off-site practice can also benefit from direct or dial-in access to the patient care system in their affiliated hospital. A 1993 survey of 133 hospitals indicated that 57 percent had a physician link with key admitters of their medical staff, and the majority were planning to expand capabilities in 1994.(15) Referring physicians enjoy having instant access to information about their hospitalized patients, and may prefer to refer patients to a hospital that provides such a service. This type of linkage will become more common as the integration of the health care industry continues.

Increasingly, physicians also find it useful to have dial-in access from their residence so they can check on patients, catch up on electronic correspondence, and do data entry; they prefer this to staying late in the hospital or having to return to do such work. The possibility of outside access raises issues of security and patient confidentiality; at the least, most hospital information systems require a second password or a callback system to ensure that the person dialing in is authorized to use the system.

Portable Access

In a classic study of physician attitudes completed in 1981, physicians rated total system portability–access at any time, from any place–as an important characteristic.(16) With the advent of hand-held devices and wireless communications, it is now much easier to provide this type of universal access. The future configuration of user devices is likely to include different types of devices in different settings. One vision is that there will be at least three classes of terminals:(17,18)

- Hand-held or ultraportable computers that are linked to the patient care system via radio frequency, used by nurses to chart patient data at the bedside, and carried routinely by residents and other physicians when they are away from their office.
- Smart terminals at nursing stations and other locations where multiple care-givers share access.
- Professional workstations, full microcomputers capable of displaying images and providing access to the patient care system, as well as to other applications and knowledge bases.

When portable devices are thoroughly integrated into patient care information systems, terminal siting issues will be simplified, costs will be reduced (due to less wiring and fewer devices needed overall), and users will have the access they need to take maximum advantage of the system.

Patient Care Information Systems Must Provide Quick and Value-Added Access to Information

Quick and Value-Added Access

As patient care information systems evolve, they capture more and more of the patient data that physicians and nurses need for patient care management. We are often inclined to measure progress in implementing clinical applications in terms of the extent to which the paper medical record is replaced with online access. This view measures progress only as increased scope of data capture and, in doing so, sells short the significant added value that patient care information systems can offer. In fact, patient care information systems can manage information proactively and provide access to patient information and views of data that go far beyond what was ever possible with paper medical records or departmental systems.

These advanced views provide many of the potential benefits of patient care information systems to direct care. This is where physicians and nurses get payback for the time they invest in entering information. The computer can present a patient-centered view, bringing together a wide range of data into a single display, or a provider-centered view, grouping all work to be done or all results from a physician's entire patient population. The computer can even use aggregate patient data to analyze clinical trends and practice patterns (as discussed in Chapter 1). This section reviews some of the design features for patient care information systems that promote quick and value-added access.

Patient-Centered Access

Once multiple types of data are available in a system and terminals and printers are located in patient care areas, physicians and nurses are generally willing to access systems themselves to retrieve patient information. Even the most basic system that makes available patient data such as laboratory and radiology results is a much more convenient and reliable repository than paper medical records. Anyone who has worked with a totally paper-based process remembers searching through incomplete medical records, telephoning the laboratory for lost or delayed results, and piecing the necessary information together from different and fragmented sources, as described in Chapter 1. Early patient care information systems that permitted nurses and physicians to inquire for patient data such as laboratory results at the nursing station could easily improve access to information as measured against this baseline.

These early systems were focused on capturing services for billing and communicating orders electronically to the work centers that needed to respond. They were designed primarily to accomplish these functions, rather than to serve as a data resource for physicians and other providers. To access results for a patient in such a system, users typically consulted one application for laboratory results, another for radiology results, and still others for admission history or other information. For each application, the user also had to sign on to the system and reidentify the patient of interest for each inquiry. Although this type of access saved time over searching through paper records and other fragmented sources of information, it had inconveniences and frustrations of its own. It did not leverage the value-added access that a patient care system can provide.

In fact, physicians rarely search for only one type of information for a patient. For both inpatients and outpatients, physicians pull together available information from several sources for each situation. Seeking multiple types of information with a traditional system meant both that users needed to initiate a large number of system queries, and that they had to record each piece of information so they could evaluate it in context. Because of the time this task required, they often turned to the unit clerk or nursing personnel to assemble system information.(19)

This method of access can be improved by minimizing the number of steps, screens, and user entries required to get to each piece of information, but cannot approach the speed or added value of patient-centered access to data. Providing patient-centered or integrated access to patient data saves both user time in obtaining needed information, and increases the value of this type of retrieval because it permits users to retrieve a set of relevant data, rather than individual data points.

With patient-centered access to clinical data the user identifies the patient of interest only once to search the database for information ranging from laboratory test results to current medication orders and latest vital signs. After identifying the patient of interest, the user also should be able to navigate easily in the system to obtain data from other types of studies and encounters. Providing the event date of the most recent result for each type of diagnostic data (radiology, chemistry, hematology, electrocardiogram, etc.) on the inquiry screen can help the user avoid futile searches for information.(20,21)

Several more advanced approaches to providing patient-centered, integrated data retrieval have also been well received by physicians because they match situations and data needs that physicians actually experience:

- A display of the most recent values for all types of diagnostic studies for a patient in a single inquiry.(22)
- An inquiry feature that allows users to query for specified types or all types of results data within a specified time frame (e.g., the last 24, 48, or 72 hours, last week).(19,23)
- The ability to request flow sheets and other displays providing multiple data points over a user-specified time period in response to a single query.(23-25)

These approaches, individually and in combination, greatly speed up the process of obtaining and compiling patient information.

Provider-Centered Access

When a physician or nurse needs access to patient information, the computer can often speed up the process by anticipating and displaying the list of patient(s) of interest. This is faster and more convenient than requiring the user to identify each patient uniquely to the system. One such patient grouping is all of the patients currently assigned to an inpatient unit (a census list).(21) When this is displayed as the default screen on terminals at a nursing station, physicians, nurses, and other providers can all easily select the patient of interest.(20) Other similar groupings are the current inpatients for whom a particular physician is the attending or a consulting physician(19), patients currently assigned to a particular nursing or clinical team, and all patients currently assigned to the service. Physicians also find it useful to maintain their own patient lists that do not fit any of the obvious standard system-maintained lists.(19,23) The current reorientation of patient management in the directions of case management and clinical pathways suggests a new grouping of patients according to the assigned case manager/interdisciplinary care team.

For ambulatory care, the most obvious grouping is patients with an appointment for a given day or clinic session. Another basis for grouping patients is those with recent outpatient encounters or admissions, the rationale being that both groups are likely to require follow-up.(26) In some settings, the ability to call up a list of most active patients or those who failed to keep appointments ("no-shows") may also be useful.(26) Other useful groupings for physician office practice are patients with outstanding telephone calls to which the physician has not yet responded(23), patients whom the physician has specifically targeted for additional contact/follow-up(27), or patients of particular interest for teaching or research(23). Managed care introduces a new useful grouping: patients assigned to a particular primary care physician/case manager. In the Emergency Department, the obvious groupings of interest to all practitioners are patients currently assigned to a particular treatment area.

Another reason that automatic patient lists are desirable is that a physician or nurse often performs the same information retrieval function on several patients in succession. In these situations the provider needs the same type of data (or data summary) for each of a defined group of patients. Examples include a resident who needs to assemble information in advance of rounds for all patients on a nursing unit, a primary care physician who needs the same type of data summary for each of the patients scheduled during a clinic session, and a nurse who needs an end-of-shift summary for each patient on the unit. Patient care information systems can facilitate system inquiries of this nature by providing multipatient access options.(24,26)

From the user's perspective, the ideal solution is the ability to place a request for a group of patients in a single system query.(19,23) To provide this type of access, a system should permit the user to designate the patient list (as discussed above) that is appropriate and then indicate what type of information is required.

In many cases, users may wish to place requests at the time they need the information ("on demand") and to indicate if they wish to review a display or printed copy. In other cases, the information required is routinely needed in the same form every day. For these repetitive requests (e.g., a summary of every patient scheduled for consultation in this clinic today), a system can be guided by predetermined rules to print the desired information at a specific time–in this case, the night before the scheduled clinic session.(23) Users can also benefit from the ability to request future printing of reports for inpatients; a resident finds it advantageous to request that up-to-date patient data summaries (rounds reports) be printed at a specific time so they are available in the morning in time for rounds.(23,24)

Much of the daily work flow for both physicians and nurses involves managing a large number of discrete tasks for a number of patients. Patient care information systems can assist in task management by identifying all patients for whom a particular care task must be performed.(28) Examples include patients with orders due to expire, patients with ordered procedures that have not been scheduled, patients with still uncharted nursing care activities during the shift, or patients with completed diagnostic procedures but no completed interpretation report. When the system can provide these task management tools on demand, it helps to ensure that all patient care tasks are attended to in a timely fashion.

Patient Views

Once there is a database rich in patient history, the value of access to historical information is enhanced by the availability of different slices through the history. Examples include:

- Chronological view: To provide insight into all information for a particular date, most recent available values for several parameters, or trends in one or more parameters over a specific period of time.
- Encounter view: Information depicting the state of knowledge about patient status at the time of a specific ambulatory encounter or admission.
- Problem-oriented view: Views of encounters and findings related to a particular disease process or problem.
- Procedure-oriented views that pull together images and text interpretation(29) or multiple images with graphical data and text.(30)

Many current hospital systems do not yet have the comprehensive database needed to provide access to all of these possible data views, especially problem- or procedure-based views. However, data for many clinically useful views can be extracted from current databases that typically include diagnostic studies, treatments, and patient measurements such as vital signs.

Physicians are often interested in trends in test results, vital signs, or other data for a particular patient over time. This can involve a large number of data points for a single or multiple patient parameters. Patient care information systems can provide views of patient data in flowsheets that display data in tabular format, graphs, histograms, nomograms, scattergrams or other formats suited to the clinical situation. The time frame of interest can be a date or date range or defined according to an event (e.g., all results since admission for this hospitalization), and users need the flexibility to identify the data, time period, and format they require.

One data view for hospitalized patients that physicians have found particularly useful is a data summary in the form of a printed rounds report.(19,24,31) This replaces the process whereby physicians collect and copy information onto index cards that they use for reference during rounds. A system-generated rounds report can be more legible and complete and is obviously a big time saver for the individual physician. Ideally, a rounds report contains information about patient problems, vital signs charted, medications administered, current orders, and completed diagnostic studies.

As the system captures a broader range of patient data, other composite views can be added to meet typical information needs, including special views suited to primary/preventive care, emergency care, and to individual clinical services such as Pediatrics and Obstetrics. Some examples include:

- "Patient at a glance" views combining clinical, visit, and demographic information about a patient.(27,32)
- Preventive medicine views, showing a wide range of health maintenance information that has been captured by the system.
- Specialist-specific views, such as flowsheets for prenatal care, arthritis functional scoring, or management of the HIV patient.
- Emergency department logs that show all patients in the department, along with their admission status, workup status, test results, and referring doctor's name.
- Discharge summaries, combining medication lists, functional assessments, and future scheduled visits.(23)

It is virtually impossible to predict exactly what information will be needed in every situation, and in what sequence. Stead et al.(28) have described the ideal access tools as a set of windows into patient data that the user can open, close, manipulate, and browse at the desired level of detail. Current patient care information systems, even those in medical informatics centers, require extensive further development before they will have tools that allow clinicians to structure their own queries in the way ideally suited to each clinical context. (These tools are likely to be provided as part of clinical workstations discussed further in the next section of this chapter).

As managed care evolves, new inquiry tools and patient views will be needed to support the new patient management roles for caregivers (addressed in Chapter

7). These will need to support preventive care more efficiently and to cover the continuum of care over longer periods of time and across settings. The new approaches to patient management are likely to increase the clinical usefulness of problem-based views of data that will permit analysis and management of the patient across both acute and ambulatory care episodes.

Management of Patient Information Review

Managing the process of reviewing patient diagnostic results is very problematic for physicians. They order multiple studies for most patients, and these often come back at different times. Managing results for inpatients is relatively easy because physicians tend to review these on a regular basis during the patient's hospital stay. For outpatients, no comparable procedures exist for checking diagnostic results; and in any case, some results are not available for days, weeks, or longer. This makes it extremely difficult for physicians to ensure that they have reviewed all of the results returned to them and followed them up when appropriate.

Particular attention must be paid to critical values, and laboratory personnel typically telephone these results to the physician or inpatient units to ensure they are received as soon as they are available. However, even this type of procedure does not always ensure that the results are communicated to the appropriate clinician in a timely fashion.(33)

Thus, in addition to managing user requests for information, patient care information systems can add value by aiding physicians and other practitioners in managing this process of reviewing and responding to patient diagnostic results. At the simplest level, this involves automatic notification concerning STAT and panic value results to the ordering physician and/or nurses station via electronic notice or automatic printing.(34) A variation on this approach is the use of digital pagers to notify nurses or physicians.(33)

Patient care information systems can aid physicians further by queuing diagnostic results through electronic mail, permitting the recipient to keep track of what he/she has reviewed. This type of system can track results not reviewed within a specified period of time, so that other measures can be taken to ensure that results are followed up.(35)

In another design, the system retains all results in the system equivalent of an electronic "in box," and users can choose to review those flagged as urgent, as well as routine results for any or all patients. Surrogate reviewers can be designated to cover for a physician as necessary, and patient care teams can be designated to all receive results for patients under their care. Users can also append comments to results or forward results to colleagues whenever appropriate.(36)

Aggregated Patient Data

When the clinical data stored in a patient care information system are highly structured, automated analysis and manipulation can serve a variety of purposes in patient care. Comprehensive patient databases themselves can serve as a knowledge base for patient care. For direct care, as well as teaching and research, clinicians can benefit from query tools that permit them to access this resource.

To the extent that useful displays and reports can be anticipated, they can be preprogrammed as standard reports. Another, more flexible approach is a user-friendly extraction tool and report generator that allows users to group patients according to clinical and/or demographic, administrative, socioeconomic attributes, and analyze differences in occurrence or variation in certain identified parameters.(34,37) In one site with a generally available clinical query tool of this type, users have access to searches based on 500 data elements. Reports can be requested by hospital administrators, as well as by physicians, residents, nurses, and medical students. Users (who completed an on-line survey following the database search) indicated that 17 percent of all requests were for patient care, 33 percent for research, 17 percent for teaching and education, 12 percent for hospital management, and 21 percent for other purposes.(37)

Sometimes users need more flexibility to structure their query. If a clinician needs to isolate a very specific subset of patients defined by a combination of more complex parameters and/or time relationships than available in a structured query tool, a more powerful and flexible query tool is required to perform unique ad hoc searches.(38) Keys to success in providing tools for searching and analyzing large clinical databases include:

- Bringing access to patient care areas so that results can potentially contribute to actual patient management.(37)
- Providing quick turnaround through a user-friendly query language that permits clinicians to access the system without the aid (and attendant delay) of programmers or other intermediaries.(5,37)
- Guiding users through the step-wise process of defining their requests, and aiding them in formulating the proper research questions.(37,38)
- Allowing users to save specifications (templates) for queries they have structured so that they can be run again as needed.
- Ensuring that use of the query tool does not negatively affect use of routine patient care applications (i.e., by impacting system performance).

The advent of patient care management according to clinical pathways brings with it new requirements for analyzing aggregated patient data across defined episodes of care. This will require not only capturing variances and reasons for variances in structured form, but also providing reports and query tools that permit differentiation of patient groups according to clinical attributes and patterns of variances. The knowledge potentially to be gained will contribute to outcomes analysis for different approaches to patient care and permit refinement of both clinical pathways and patient assignment to clinical pathways.

Access to Knowledge Resources

In addition to patient data, patient care information systems can provide other information that physicians need through access to reference materials and bibliographic databases. This information can potentially be consulted as needed for specific patients at the point of care, and it can also help physicians and nurses keep abreast of new developments that affect their practice areas.

Online access to the medical literature through current patient care information systems is most often described as an adjunct to research and teaching in teaching hospitals. One study of the information needs that arise during clinical teaching revealed that 26 percent of the questions that arise during rounds require reference to a textbook or the medical literature.(39) High rates of use have been reported when physicians and other users in an academic medical center are given access to search the medical literature through a clinical information system that links them to an online bibliographic database and a program that guides the user in framing a search strategy.(40) General practice physicians have also indicated in several surveys that they feel online access to the medical literature would improve their ability to practice medicine(41,42), and one of the stated goals for the computer-based record system is to bring access to medical knowledge to the point of care in any setting.(2)

In their study of questions that arise during rounds in a teaching hospital, Osheroff et al.(39) reported that most questions that could be answered using the medical literature were posed in patient-specific terms, and required locating information that fit a very specific clinical problem. For a bibliographic database to provide clinically relevant information, its search algorithm must compose the right question. Initial results of one study of practicing physicians indicated that accessing the medical literature provided relevant information to the questions that arise in primary care practice only 58 percent of the time, and a clear answer only 46 percent of the time.(43) This illustrates the challenge of matching specific clinical information needs with the relevant information resources. Current research in a number of informatics centers is geared to developing domain-specific query tools and knowledge bases that will provide context-sensitive, patient-centered access to information resources, thereby maximizing the value of this access for patient management.(44-48)

In addition to the medical literature, other types of information resources can be useful for practicing physicians.(49) For example, when physicians can review the frequently consulted *Physicians' Desk Reference* online they save time in locating a copy when they need it and are also able to consult the latest edition. Other decision support tools that are routinely consulted include information concerning drug-drug, drug-test, and drug-problem interactions, and programs that provide assistance with complicated calculations.(34,49)

Patient Care Information Systems Must Be Designed to Fit Actual Patient Care Processes and Work Situations

Fit with Clinical Environment

If patient care information systems are to be incorporated as an information resource partner in routine care processes, they must fit the environment in which physicians, nurses, and other users work. The RAND study of interactive information systems in the general office setting concluded that the extent to which applications suit the routine tasks of users is a good predictor of success in voluntary incorporation into day-to-day work.(50) The lack of acceptance of early order communication/results reporting systems by physicians in particular can be explained largely because these systems were designed primarily to fit billing and ancillary department processes rather than the clinical work environment.

Accumulated experience with advanced patient care information systems also validates the importance of design driven by a detailed understanding of patient care processes. Achieving fit with these processes requires considering many different dimensions. First, applications need to address processes rather than individual, unrelated tasks. The best example of this is order entry. Designs for early attempts to engage physicians in entering their orders generally treated this as a stand-alone function. In practice, physicians usually evaluate and change patient orders as part of the larger process of assessing/reassessing patient status and progress and developing the care strategy. Although writing orders is one task within this process, it is intermingled with reviewing current orders, checking for diagnostic results, and examining trends in status indicators such as patient vital signs. To be incorporated successfully into this process, a patient care system must allow the user to perform all of these tasks in any sequence and move easily and quickly from one to the next.

Another aspect of fit requires taking the actual work environment into account. For example, interruptions are one notable feature of the work environment of the house officer.(51) One time-motion study of internal medicine interns found that they were paged two times an hour during the day and spent a mean of only 2.4 minutes on an activity before being interrupted.(52) Another time study of internal medicine house staff on call in three different hospitals found that staff received 16 to 25 pages and 13 to 39 telephone calls per night, and the mean time before a history/physical examination for a new patient was interrupted was 7 to 11 minutes.(51) The implications for system design are that users should be able to terminate a user session very quickly and, especially when engaged in data entry, restart in the same function or task exactly where they were working when they were interrupted.

Patient Care Scenarios

The computer in the clinical setting is only a tool, and the fundamental activity of care delivery is the personal interaction of physicians, nurses, and other caregivers with patients. These person-to-person interactions take a large number of forms in different care settings and domains of clinical practice, and each of these has its own information process.

The complexity and variety of patient care scenarios can be illustrated by one example from a design effort to create a primary care ambulatory practice record.(27) System designers have identified the following major patient scenarios:

- Physician's morning preparation in advance of the clinic session, including review of active problems and preventive care considerations for patients scheduled to be seen.
- Initial visit between patient and provider.
- Follow-up visit, for new or old problems.
- Physician response to a telephone call from a patient.
- Patient encounter with other providers for specific tasks (e.g., dose adjustment for warfarin).
- Patient visit to consultant or Emergency Department.
- Review of pending studies and work to be done between visits.

Since each of these has a unique flow of information requirements, the next step is to determine the exact work flow of each, including what data are needed, what data are interrelated, and how data-related tasks are likely to be sequenced.

This type of careful examination of patient care scenarios allows the designer to develop the specialized views of patient data tailored to the care situation (as discussed further under *Value-Added Access to Information*) and provide easy ways for the user to move among tasks so that the system interaction is compatible with the actual work flow. In some cases, the system may be able to give added value by automatically providing the information most likely to be needed next or by offering to facilitate entering orders or initiating communication with other care providers (e.g., offering to send a message to the intake nurse that this patient needs an influenza vaccination).

The variety and complexity of patient care scenarios are daunting. Some designers have conducted ethnographic studies of information-creating and seeking behavior in different care scenarios to provide the direction for basic design of advanced clinical applications and work stations.(39,53-55) The challenge of addressing actual patient care scenarios has also led to the substantial involvement of users in the design effort through prototyping and/or pilot testing to expand the understanding of needs and the appropriateness of solutions.(5,56,57) (This approach has also been recommended for the implementation/tailoring of advanced patient care information systems purchased from vendors[17,58]). Several developers have recommended monitoring system use (through special system monitoring tools built into the system and/or observation) as an effective means of obtaining feedback concerning what users are accessing functions and the volumes of use.(19,22,59) This can supplement the information gained through observation and discussions with users about the extent to which their needs are being addressed.

An example of how a variety of tasks can be combined in a way that is compatible with the actual patient care process is provided by one design for support to telephone consultation:(23,36)

- Patient messages can be recorded in the system by the physician or designated others such as secretary, triage nurse, etc. Each call is maintained online in incomplete status until the physician notes that it has been addressed, and multiple attempts to contact the patient (as well as repeat calls from the patient) are recorded as part of the same record.
- The basic screen for viewing during the telephone consultation incorporates patient demographics and telephone contact information, and users can request a recent activity summary from the same screen. Physicians can record a simple note to document the conversation and forward completed notes to medical records, other colleagues, or their own electronic mailboxes for future referral.

By combining the tasks of tracking patient calls, retrieving patient information to contact the patient and address the case in question, and documenting the interaction, this design is intended to be compatible with the actual process as it occurs in the physician office, including contributions of and communication with other involved personnel.

System Flexibility

Clinical practices in different health care delivery organizations are likely to have established very different patterns of information use. Designers of systems intended for widespread distribution within and among institutions must have an approach to support all of these practices, without exhausting themselves by trying to anticipate and customize each one.

In fact, there is substantial common ground in basic processes and clinical domains that can be addressed by the same work flow models. However, additional features–dictated by local interest or policy, differences in patient populations, and possibly research–will always need to be incorporated if the patient care information system is to achieve its greatest potential contribution to patient information management. For example, physicians in a rheumatology practice may want to use a flow sheet for pain and mobility scores; a prenatal clinic may want special features for entry and review of weight, fundal height, heart rate, and urinalysis. One way to accommodate such needs is through a flexible system that permits users to design screen content and flow for such applications.

Another strong rationale for flexibility in patient care information systems is changes in models for care delivery and management such as case/episode management, patient-focused care, and clinical pathways. As discussed in Chapter 7, these are changing both the roles and approaches of members of the care delivery team and bring new requirements for assembling and evaluating patient information. As institutions phase in these new approaches, they will need the ability to implement them selectively to gain experience, while retaining more traditional approaches in many areas.

Flexible systems can be difficult to build; the designer is effectively ceding some control over the operation of the system to a person who may be unskilled in computer programming. Systems must be protected against programming errors that would corrupt the database or crash the system. Another challenge is making user tools easy to operate. The tools must draw the elements of screens to meet the local needs and match screen elements to the proper items in the system's data dictionary.

Nonetheless, systems can often be user-customizable to handle a multitude of different custom clinical information scenarios. Most commercial database programs have some sort of query and form-design capability, requiring only a limited amount of training before users can operate these effectively. An increasing number of commercial patient care information systems provide screen-design capability. Companies designing such systems often work with their users to accumulate a large set of pre-fabricated screen layouts, that can be distributed to other customer sites as a starter kit. Similar approaches are likely to be used to enable site definition and tailoring of clinical pathways as these are released in commercial products.

Flexibility should also extend to prompts, reminders, and other applications that combine medical knowledge and logic with patient data. As discussed in Chapter 1, there are now many examples of these applications and information on their potential contributions to patient care. Most of the published work, however, has come from settings where the clinical applications are designed and programmed locally. This means that the local medical staff can structure the logic, as well as the nature and style of the system advice; it appears that this aids both initial buy-in and clinical utility. Over time, as knowledge about applying decision support increases and the databases in patient care information systems become richer, the flexibility to refine and extend these applications will remain important.

The ultimate in flexibility is user customization. For office-based systems, Bikson et al.(50) found that user modifiability makes a substantial contribution to user satisfaction. For patient care information systems as well, there is increasing evidence that acceptance can be enhanced when users are able to customize system features to suit their individual preferences. In one center, for example, physician users of a system featuring a data summary for inpatients were permitted to define their own template for this summary, specifying the type and sequence of data fields, the time order, and time period to be displayed. After the self-customization feature had been available for only 6 weeks, users requested customized reports 51 percent of the time.(19)

Customization to suit individual needs and preferences is one of the major design goals for the new model of the physician professional workstation that is intended to provide a more intuitive and flexible front-end for patient care applications.(60,61) Users of these workstations may be able to control the look of the screen (icons or pictures used to identify data types and functions, data sequence, field placement and appearance, color, etc.), as well as the manner in which they are notified of reminders, alerts, and priority messages.(62)

In thinking about the potential contributions of advanced workstations to user efficiency and acceptance, it is important to differentiate format from content.(63) Although workstations will undoubtedly further increase ease of use and flexibility, a number of authors have cautioned that there are examples of advanced patient care information systems based on dumb terminals that have achieved user acceptance based on the value of information content.(34,64,65) Features of the successful workstation will also need to reflect careful attention to the different information needs of each group of professional caregivers who will use it.(66)

Patient Care Information Systems Must Be So Easy to Use That They Require Little (or No) Training

Importance of Minimizing Training

Physicians and nurses are less likely to accept a new clinical system if it requires extensive training before they can become proficient users. A heavy requirement for training can prejudice potential users against the system from the outset. It is also undesirable for several practical reasons.

The most obvious problem with training is that there is no time to do it. Rearranging patient care responsibilities in order to accommodate training is likely to reduce productivity; paying overtime in order to do off-shift training can be very costly. Conducting training during unpaid overtime is inadvisable. The situation is still more difficult when private-practice physicians are expected to devote time away from their practice for system training.

In teaching hospitals, it is impractical to expect each group of new residents or medical students to attend lengthy training sessions before they can begin their work as they are likely to need to begin caring for patients almost immediately.(59) In this setting, training time of more than an hour, or a learning curve of more than a day or two, is unrealistic.(56) High rates of turnover among nurses and the need to employ contract nurses in many hospitals can also increase the number of staff to be trained.

The costs of formal training are increased if the patient care information system is being implemented in phases, requiring physicians and nurses to master several different ways of using the system. (Alternate approaches to implementation are discussed in Chapter 6.) Periodic enhancements to the system also increase this burden if they necessitate extra instruction.

Even more importantly, extensive training is not a propitious beginning for a patient care information systems venture in which many of the users are likely to be reluctant participants, at best. Many of the potential users of patient care information systems own or have worked with personal computers. They expect to be able to master the functions they need to use in any other system with relative speed and effort. When this turns out not to be the case, they are likely to conclude that the new tool is unnecessarily difficult to master and, therefore, inadequate.(67)

For all of these reasons, a stated design objective of many systems is that there should be no need of formal training for physicians and other users of clinical functions.(20,22,56,59,65,68) To make this possible, systems must be as intuitive and easy to use as possible. This sets a very high standard for patient care information systems in general. However, it is an attainable goal, and many clinical applications involving physicians and nurses as direct users have been implemented under this guideline.

Intuitive Design to Reduce Memory Burden

Ease of use can be translated into specific design features at several different levels. One way to characterize ease of use is the memory burden required for users to understand the system. Ideally, even the novice computer user should feel there is no specialized vocabulary or procedure to master. This is especially true for physician users who are likely to call up some clinical applications only infrequently. Many staff physicians in teaching hospitals fit this category, as do private practice physicians in community hospitals who may admit patients to several different hospitals.

Sporadic users will have greater difficulty mastering and remembering complex procedures for entering and retrieving data, compared with residents and other staff who use the system more intensively. In one teaching hospital in which we have worked, residents were responsible for inpatient order entry in the system. Many staff physicians concluded that they could not master the system's order entry process, which involved many system pathways, steps, and function keys. Because they were not confident that they could enter the necessary orders correctly, they announced that they could no longer take weekend rotations to spell the residents as they had done in the past.

In many cases, physician use of clinical functions is voluntary and, unless they conclude that the system is a reasonable tool, they simply will not use it.

This was the case in one academic medical center, where physicians who found a computerized ambulatory medical record confusing reportedly quit using the system altogether.(69) In one trial of order entry by nurses in which system use was required, users who felt the system was confusing were less likely to enter data in a timely fashion.(70)

Terminology

Systems are easier to use if the terminology is familiar. For clinical applications, this means that medical terminology should match the terms that physicians and nurses use in practice. When they are requesting patient data or identifying a service they need to order, they should select or enter an item that makes sense to them rather than have to remember an otherwise unfamiliar term required by the system. When multiple synonyms for the same concept are routinely used, patient care information systems should understand all of these. For example, physicians often use abbreviations or short forms: TNG for nitroglycerin, T4 for thyroxine. Considerable fine-tuning of these terms can be required to match them to all of the variations in practice.

Prompts and Cues

When users need to perform computer tasks, prompts and on-screen cues should be understandable and instructional. An important element of making a system easy to use is to ensure that even first-time users can follow instructions and understand each on-screen cue or choice so that learning time is minimized.(71) The process for getting into and out of each function and application should be obvious. Likewise, when data entries fail validity checks, or when users otherwise attempt some function that occasions a system error, the error message should clearly instruct the user in how to rectify the problem.

Single Interface

Learning time can be minimized if users feel they are mastering one, unified system that looks and feels the same throughout the range of functions they use. In fact, patient care information systems may draw data from multiple underlying ancillary department systems: one for laboratory data, another for information on drug orders, a third for a patient's history of admissions or outpatient encounters. Users will not feel that the system is easy to use if they have to learn a different way of interacting with each application to get their work done. Standardized prompts and user entries, consistent screen design and navigational aids, even consistent use of color all contribute to giving the user only one system to learn.

Online Help

An easy, consistent interface with understandable terminology will contribute to users' comfort and confidence. So will the presence of readily available online help. Sooner or later a user will encounter a task that he or she does not understand fully. If help is immediately available from the computer itself, the user does not need to take the time to call a systems operator and wait for a response.

Online help can take the form of one- or two-line instruction fields placed right on the clinical screens, and/or full help screens describing the functions in more detail. Each help screen should be clearly written and should be context-sensitive (i.e., targeted to the specific function the user is trying to perform).

Some centers have developed online tutorials. Although these can be time-consuming to develop, they can provide rewards, even when the system is generally easy to operate. Users can practice with the tutorial in spare moments when they need to review the use of the computer; this can be especially beneficial when there are many occasional or infrequent users.

Range of Users

Groups of users of patient care information systems typically include both extremely computer literate users who may have even done their own programming and total novices who are intimidated by the prospect of using a system. Providing systems that are considered easy to use by such a broad range of users is a double challenge.

Novice users need to be guided so that they easily accomplish their tasks; more expert users are likely to look for shortcuts such as user-defined keys or macro routines that allow them to complete the desired operation as quickly as possible. They may also seek ways to customize the system to their personal preferences.

Novice users may become more competent in computer tasks. However, we have found that many physicians are far more interested in quickly incorporating effective and efficient information tools into their practice than they are in learning to become computer experts. Once they decide that a system is worth learning, they learn whatever they feel is necessary to become efficient at meeting their needs and settle quickly into their adopted mode of accomplishing system tasks. The quicker they are able to do so, the more likely they are to accept and use the system routinely. This increases the importance of "doing it right the first time."

Involving Physicians with Direct Entry Requires Minimizing Time and Maximizing Incentives

Need for Direct Entry

Physicians and nurses are the authors, as well as the users, of much of the information captured in medical records. Patient information created by clinicians is ideally entered in the computer by its originator at the point of service.(2,72,73) This approach can increase timeliness and accuracy, and eliminate the cost of clerical intermediaries. In addition, as discussed in Chapter 1, alerts and warnings generated by advanced patient care information systems are often triggered by new orders (for example, drug interactions related to a new medication order), and they affect the patient's subsequent orders and interventions. If the orders are entered on the computer by the physician, the alerts can be presented at the very time they are needed in the physician's planning process. Thus, there are sufficient reasons to encourage physicians to enter data directly into the computer, if direct entry does not impede their ability to provide care. We believe that meeting this challenge requires providing systems with user interactions that are as close as possible to time neutral and add as much information value as possible as an incentive.

Minimizing Time

Health care professionals operate under considerable time constraints. Physicians and nurses with whom we work typically cite time pressures as one of their biggest problems and time management as one of their biggest challenges. Not surprisingly, they are reluctant to learn and adapt to any system that they believe takes them longer to accomplish their work. Looking at this issue from another perspective, the challenge for the system developer is to make patient care information systems easier to use than not to use(74) or with benefits that outweigh the user effort.(75)

Ideally, the computer saves time with each task a user performs on the system and this is an important design objective for system developers.(5,76-78) As we move toward more advanced patient care information systems and eventually computer-based patient records, systems should make both data retrieval *and* data entry more efficient. Systems to date have generally succeeded in making information retrieval more efficient. They have usually faltered, however, in engaging physicians in direct entry because the system was originally designed for clerk entry and physicians find the alternative of pen and paper much quicker and more straightforward.

According to the Institute of Medicine study, "perhaps the single greatest challenge that has consistently confronted every clinical system developer is to engage clinicians in direct entry."(2) A number of sentinel, self-developed patient care information systems are designed for physician direct entry of some types of data.(79) Some commercial hospital information systems offer the capability for physician order entry, while medical record systems such as COSTAR can engage physicians in documenting patient problems and notes directly in the system. However, many reports in the field describe failed efforts to engage physicians in entering patient orders in particular.(80) The literature on direct entry, both successes and failures, comes mainly from academic medical centers with medical informatics programs or from custom systems used in individual practices or clinics; even in these settings, 100 percent physician acceptance is rare.

System developers/implementors have a tendency to view time savings gained for patient data retrieval as an offset to any extra user time that may be needed for data entry tasks. Certainly, if one evaluates the impact (or potential impact) of a patient care system on *total user time,* savings in information retrieval efficiency are likely to outweigh increased time devoted to direct entry of orders and documentation. In our experience, however, physicians are more inclined to view these tasks separately and to expect data entry as well to be at least time neutral. Gains and losses in efficiency are usually very apparent to physicians and other users because patient care support is usually phased in, with results retrieval preceding more advanced functions. Therefore, by the time physicians are presented with the opportunity for direct entry, they have normally assimilated the ease of system results retrieval into their routine and do not perceive entry and retrieval as a package deal.

Order Entry

Orders are the logical first step in engaging physicians in direct entry because there are significant benefits to timeliness and accuracy, and because orders are simpler to automate than physician documentation such as history/physical and progress notes. A computer needs structured information to interpret each order correctly, however. This requires a degree of standardization never achieved with handwritten orders, and it complicates the challenge of making system order entry as easy as the pen and paper process it replaces. Consequently, success with physician order entry is viewed as an "acid test" for any patient care information system.(81)

We believe that physician opposition to order entry has been based on the time required, rather than an inherent aversion to performing this function. Most of the published reports come from teaching hospitals and involve interns or residents entering orders for inpatients. Physicians are accustomed to writing inpatient orders in a brief and sometimes cryptic manner; because of this history, it is very difficult to design system order entry without increasing physician time substantially. In one published report involving order entry with a commercial patient care information system, residents rotating on some order-intensive services spent more than 2 hours on the system each day.(67) In one teaching hospital in which the clinical system designers focused on achieving an acceptable physician interface, a time-motion study indicated that interns spent 80 percent more time entering admission orders, and 200 percent more time to enter daily orders into the system than their colleagues.(82)

One of the keys to improving the speed of order entry is to permit entry of order parameters in a familiar sequence and format. This includes the ability to enter any mix of order types rather than having to access a separate module or pathway for medications, laboratory, etc. Another key to success is to require only the information a physician is accustomed to providing in an order, not all of the other details such as routine scheduling of "q-shift" tasks on the nursing unit or specific base fluids to use in IV admixtures. The design for physician inpatient order entry should take into account the many variations in frequency and pattern of administration that exist for medication orders, including sliding scales, tapers, and alternate-day dosing. For each of these types of orders, special routines are needed to permit users to enter interpretable orders efficiently.

Order sets can significantly shorten the time needed to enter orders. System order sets are the equivalent of written protocols for a particular event (e.g., admission for a given diagnosis) or clinical situation (e.g., postprocedure orders for patients with uneventful surgery), which are already used routinely in many care situations. They provide a starting point for the physician to consider any modifications needed for the particular patient. A department can establish official order sets; these can aid the implementation of departmental standards. In our experience, physicians who utilize order sets report time savings over entering orders individually. However, order sets apply most readily to a limited number of clinical situations; they do not solve the entire problem of ordering time.

Another approach that works on the same principle is to allow each physician to store orders for the most frequently ordered medications, diagnostic tests, and other services in a "favorites list." The physician can then select and sign one or more orders applicable to any new patient. This approach is potentially useful for many types of outpatient practice, where physicians see a large number of patients with similar problems. Many physicians we have interviewed believe that they could enter as many as 70 to 80 percent of their outpatient orders via this mechanism.

When combined with outpatient scheduling, a further enhancement to order sets and the "favorites list" would pull the appropriate list of possible orders based on the patient's appointment type (e.g., annual physical). As patient care information systems become more advanced and incorporate embedded knowledge, systems will be able to suggest orders based on combinations of patient characteristics (e.g., age, diagnosis) and applicable guidelines or protocols.

(The experience with physician order entry at the Brigham and Women's Hospital is described at the end of this chapter.)

Patient Documentation

Compared with order entry, there have been many fewer attempts at getting physicians to enter documentation: history and physical, encounter and progress notes, discharge summaries, and operative reports. These are probably a bigger challenge because orders lend themselves more readily to the structured format the system requires than do free-text notes.

Physicians generally dictate large texts such as discharge summaries and operative notes. A transcriptionist uses a word processor to copy dictation; the resulting text file can be copied directly into the system database, where the clinician can review and electronically sign it. For shorter notes, the computer system can display forms that are familiar to nurses and physicians and easy to use. In trials, this method has eased the transition to the computer and reduced time, compared with an approach based on pull-down menus.(76,83)

Physicians and nurses are accustomed to handwriting (or dictating) a freeform narrative in documenting care. Most computerized record systems store the actual text, without conversion. If the notes are to be useful for reporting and decision support applications, they must be entered in a structured fashion, with defined vocabularies. Structured entry based on menus and user selection of choices works best if the choices for a given field can be narrowly defined and displayed in a short list or on a single screen. This approach can work if the particular practice uses a well-constrained scope of information, as in a specialty practice or a radiology group. For a primary-care practice's encounter notes, there would be far too many choices to display. Further advances in continuous-speech voice recognition and language processors to transform free text into coded data will be needed before it will be feasible for physicians to enter structured information of this type as a general practice. Some work has been done commercially with systems for emergency medicine (Kurzweil, CIAI, IBM), although these usually work better for relatively uncomplicated patient encounters.

Data entry time can be reduced when the system prompts with the most likely response whenever possible. In some cases, the ability to carry over previous entries with only minor editing can decrease user time. One example is a system that copies physician-entered discharge summary information to incorporate into a nursing discharge summary(23, 84); another system imports information from the nurse's note from the prior shift as the starting point for nurse charting.(85) It is vitally important, however, that clinicians who use this method carefully review the imported information to be sure that it reflects their own impressions of the patient and have efficient ways to edit or replace information that does not pertain. Another recent effort to speed up the process of creating structured progress notes relies upon clinical findings to prompt entries.(86)

Entry of patient problem lists is an easier task than entry of full text. Problems are typically only a few words long, and thus are easier for users to enter. Problem lists offer potential benefits to care because they convey important knowledge about the patient (in one project involving a computerized ambulatory record, 46 percent of user accesses involved retrieval of the patient problem list[87]). However, a lack of standard terminology makes it difficult to create coded problem lists from typical user entries. Several centers have worked toward the creation of standard problem codes.(88-91) One experimental approach with the HELP System involves a number of different keyword and phrase matching algorithms to reduce user keystrokes and achieve coded input.(92)

There is a critical-mass effect to data entry. As more data are entered into the system, it is more likely that a physician looking for information will find it on the computer; thus, the physician is more likely to continue to support the system. Physicians using one electronic outpatient medical record were initially reluctant to use the system, until other staff provided assistance by entering existing initial problem and medication lists from paper charts, so that physicians only needed to enter updates. The physicians grew increasingly amenable to maintaining problem and medication lists themselves as the value of the online data increased.(93)

Modes of Entry

If physicians, nurses, and other users are to interact routinely with patient care information systems, they should be comfortable and proficient with the mode of entering or requesting information.

Since keyboard entry remains the predominant mode, physician reluctance to interact with systems has sometimes been attributed to an inability or unwillingness to type. In an informal survey of physicians and residents in one teaching hospital, we found that two thirds rated themselves as reasonably proficient typists, and only 11 percent rated themselves as "slow hunt and peck" typists. A recent survey conducted in an HMO that was implementing an outpatient information system revealed that 69 percent had learned to touch type. (94) Although keyboard entry may still be a barrier for some potential users, we believe the critical factor for most is time rather than a disinclination to type. In one trial of a clinic electronic record, for example, researchers concluded that typing was not a barrier to physician entry of problem lists and found that physicians tend to type longer notes than they dictate.(93,95)

Alternatives such as pointing devices (light pen, mouse, track ball) for item selection, now common in other computer applications, have been incorporated into some current patient care information systems. Some users report that using a mouse is tiring and that the necessary surface area is not always available in patient care areas. Light pens and touch screens have been criticized because they are too expensive and do not permit displaying as many user selections on a screen.(92,96) Although no single method is clearly preferable, some reports indicate that many users actually prefer keyboard entry, especially those accustomed to using a system routinely.(13,35,97)

New technology offers alternatives that appear to be well suited for some data entry situations. Voice recognition has been applied to physician reporting traditionally done by dictation–radiology, pathology, and emergency medicine–but more recently to nursing progress notes as well.(98) When combined with domain-specific prompting and standardized entry, voice recognition can provide structured data, not achieved with traditional dictation, in some circumstances.

Pen-based computing has been applied successfully to nurse charting, where nurses could check off tasks and findings on a form, with any comments entered via handwriting.(76) Handwriting recognition is still an inconsistent technology at this time, however, and further development is required to improve pen-based input before it can become a routine input modality.(99) In one comparison of multiple modes for nurse entry of numerical data in the ICU setting, a graphics tablet with an application-specific overlay was faster and resulted in more accurate data entry than more traditional modes such as keyboard and mouse or cursor keys with drop-down menus.(100)

Eventually, as physicians and other users enter more patient data into patient care information systems, they are likely to require that multiple modes be available, to suit both individual preferences and differing data entry tasks and settings.(101,102)

Extra Incentives

A number of system incentives can be incorporated into patient care information systems to increase the motivation for data entry. If the system task itself is not time neutral, then it is important that the cost to benefit ratio for the clinical user not be increased.(101) One way of offsetting time increases and/or increasing motivation is to provide immediate tangible benefits to the user.

Physicians and nurses will have more incentive to perform data entry if the entered data can save them work and provide benefits in other areas. A prime example of this is a project involving resident-entered discharge summaries. When these were completed the night prior to discharge, the system would prepare a set of filled out discharge prescriptions for the resident to sign, complete the physician portion of the discharge form, and provide a printed summary that could be used for referral to another facility. Because nurses could obtain printed patient medication instructions and avoid preparing interagency referral forms, they encouraged the residents to prepare their summaries online.(103) Current examples include systems that provide printed prescriptions as an incentive for a physician to enter outpatient medications. An added benefit of such a system is its ability to renew a prescription with minimal effort.(35)

Other incentives are based on providing efficient and timely means of communicating with colleagues. In one hospital, completed discharge summaries, operative reports, and diagnostic procedure reports are automatically sent to referring physicians in other institutions via an electronic mail link.(34) In another site, physicians who enter notes online can send copies via electronic mail to the referring physician or another colleague involved in the care of the patient.(23)

Some of the most direct and tangible incentives are financial. In the same project involving discharge summaries discussed above, residents were offered $5 by the hospital for each summary completed in the system. This not only resulted in a net savings to the hospital over the cost of transcription, but also provided other advantages such as timely completion and signature.(68) Examples have now been reported of physicians negotiating reductions in malpractice premiums in exchange for using system order sets and printed discharge instructions(104) and directly entering structured patient reports for patients seen in an emergency room.(105)

Clinical Pathways

New case management techniques such as clinical pathways promise to make the entry of assessments, orders, and progress notes much easier. As discussed in Chapter 7, a clinical pathway is a map of the anticipated sequence and timing of interventions and assessments for a particular diagnosis or procedure. Originally applied to nursing case management(106), clinical pathways have become interdisciplinary, reflecting care plans and results for all members of a care team, from physician and nurse to respiratory therapist and social worker.(107)

Each clinical pathway is developed jointly by members of the various disciplines involved in the case. It provides an agreed-upon "typical" clinical course against which the team manages patient care episodes. For each defined time period, the clinical pathway contains specific interventions such as diagnostic studies, medications, nursing care, and consults, anticipated patient status and progress. Nursing and physician members of the care team can view the anticipated interventions for each time period and use these as a starting point in designing the care plan, accepting those that fit the patient and making necessary revisions. (This is analogous to the use of order sets and templates for nursing care plans.) Anticipated outcomes for each time period in the clinical path can also be displayed, reviewed, and signed.(108)

Charting by exception, a documentation concept used primarily for inpatient nursing, displays nursing tasks and normal findings for the nurse to check off and sign (electronically if implemented on a system) and requires the nurse only to annotate significant findings, exceptions to norms, or tasks not completed. (109) Charting by exception has been successfully incorporated into current nursing systems and many patient care information systems. Clinical pathways include the expected improvements in patient outcome for each time period, as well as the orders for all services and interventions. If these are all set up in the patient care system, assuming that a patient's clinical course is as anticipated, all members of the care team can place orders and enter observations in this manner, instead of having to create or select each entry individually. When a variance or detour from the clinical pathway occurs, the cause must be entered in coded form so that the system can provide reports for use in variance analysis. In addition to providing consistent, structured data that can be aggregated for management reporting and research, this approach can make ordering, charting, and note writing significantly quicker than accomplishing these tasks on paper.

Clinical pathways have been initially applied to in-hospital care, but are being extended to prehospital and postdischarge care and are likely to be used eventually to manage patients over extended periods of time and across institutional settings.(110) In most health care organizations, only a limited number of clinical pathways are currently being developed or implemented because of the significant coordination and time required to develop and implement them. In most cases, system support to apply clinical pathways efficiently to large numbers of patients and diagnoses is also not yet available.(111) However, this innovation in patient management, combined with appropriate support from patient care information systems, offers great potential to optimize the information management tasks of both physicians and nurses and successfully engage both groups of users in direct system interaction.

Examples from BICS

Overview

Brigham and Women's Hospital (BWH) in Boston is a 750-bed urban teaching hospital, serving both its local community and a tertiary referral population. The Brigham Integrated Computing System (BICS) at BWH is a large computing network, which is used by nearly every department in the hospital.(112) BICS was originally derived from the hospital computing system at Beth Israel Hospital (22); many central functions from the original system are still in operation. Starting in 1988, as BWH continued to grow, the Information Systems Department converted the computer system to run on a microcomputer network for increased power and flexibility. Independent development of software at BWH for the new system has continued since that time. The hospital now has more than 3,000 workstations.

Many of the principles described earlier in this chapter have been used to develop clinical applications on BICS. BICS is used every day by nurses, doctors, and other clinical professionals; these users perform data retrieval and data entry on a regular basis. Physicians enter data for inpatient orders, the ambulatory record, patient summaries, and related applications; nurses perform entry for orders, bed management, patient acuity scoring, and other functions. This section describes some of the major subsystems developed for BICS, in the context of the design principles defined in this chapter: improved organization of data, accessibility wherever and whenever it is needed, value-added features provided, its ability to support typical clinical scenarios, the incentives for data entry, and features for general ease of use.

General System

BICS is available 24 hours a day. Formerly, the system had 1 to 2 hours of scheduled downtime for backup, three times a week. In the current microcomputer network, all data are stored in duplicate: the primary server runs continuously, while the system backup is taken from the secondary ("ghost") server. When this process is completed, the ghost catches up on the data that is added during the backup. In case of a failure in the primary server, the ghost can cut in and provide continuous service. An uninterruptible power supply protects the servers from brownouts and power failures.

Workstations are located on all inpatient floors, in all ambulatory practices, most business offices, and in other strategic locations such as the library. On inpatient units there are five workstations per 15-bed unit; in intensive-care areas one station serves one or two beds. Dedicated copper and fiber-optic cable connects off-site facilities and clinical sites of the hospital's primary HMO. Users who have demonstrated need can sign on to the system from outside of the hospital via modem. An extra password is required for remote access. Otherwise, remote operation looks the same as on-site operation, including the use of pointing devices.

New BICS applications use a windowed user interface (Hyper-M), which can be controlled from the keyboard or from a pointing device such as a mouse. System controls, colors, and names on command buttons are standardized to give all programs a similar look and feel. Most clinical-systems programs are developed in cooperation with a group of eventual users of the new programs. Members of the users' group help to specify the desired functions of the programs, then test them for utility and ease of use before the program is released.

Formal training in the use of the system is minimal. Physicians receive a 45-minute group introduction to order entry and basic system operation; after this, they use the system independently. Nurses receive a similar amount of training.

Ambulatory Record

The BICS ambulatory record has been adopted in the primary care medicine practice and in several other outpatient practices.(27) The record serves as a replacement for the paper chart. The ambulatory record contains problem lists, progress notes (chronological and problem-oriented), medications and allergies, vital signs, pending "to do" items, and health maintenance information. Laboratory results, discharge summaries, and all other online clinical information can be viewed as well. Workstations are located in intake areas, in examination rooms, and in physician offices. The system has been operating in essentially unchanged form since 1989.

The record is designed to support the most frequent clinical scenarios, as discussed earlier in this chapter. The patient summary screen (Figure 4-1) provides a "patient-at-a-glance" view of problems, medications, allergies, and recent visits; this screen is of particular interest to the physician who needs a general summary or overview of a new patient. From this screen, the user can branch out to get more detail in any of the data categories noted in the preceding paragraph.

A physician in the BWH Emergency Department, seeking information on an unfamiliar patient, typically checks first to see if recent discharge summaries exist. After this, the physician normally looks up the patient's ambulatory record for a summary, then reads the recent progress notes.

For the physician who knows the patient well, the "day-at-a glance" view (Figure 4-2) gives a record of all of the data produced at the last visit and any other recent visits to other providers. This view shows the visit date and provider, the diagnoses for the visit, and a list of the available data–for example, "NCHEkg" indicates that a progress note, chemistry and hematology laboratory values, and an electrocardiogram are filed for this visit. By choosing the visit number, the user can see all of these data immediately.

The primary value of the BICS ambulatory record is that it is available at any time, at any location, and that any particular type of data is always found in the same section. No special training is required for physicians to learn to use the ambulatory record because the record follows the same interface standards as the rest of the system. Administrative costs are reduced because the paper record does not have to be retrieved, collated, and refiled.

In addition, several features give added value to users of the record. The day-at-a-glance view combines all information relating to the visit, regardless of when data (such as laboratory results) may have been entered. The health maintenance

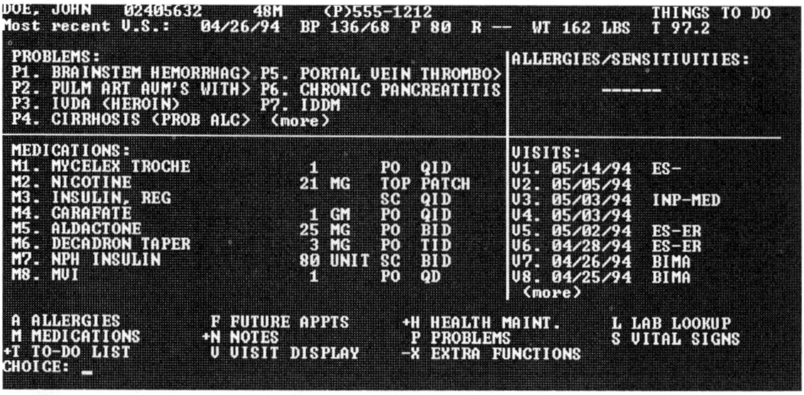

```
DOE, JOHN      02405632    48M    (P)555-1212                     THINGS TO DO
Most recent V.S.:    04/26/94  BP 136/68  P 80  R --  WT 162 LBS  T 97.2

PROBLEMS:                                    ALLERGIES/SENSITIVITIES:
P1. BRAINSTEM HEMORRHAG> P5. PORTAL VEIN THROMBO>
P2. PULM ART AUM'S WITH> P6. CHRONIC PANCREATITIS
P3. IVDA (HEROIN>        P7. IDDM             ----
P4. CIRRHOSIS (PROB ALC> (more)

MEDICATIONS:                                 VISITS:
M1. MYCELEX TROCHE            1       PO  QID  V1. 05/14/94  ES-
M2. NICOTINE                21 MG   TOP PATCH  V2. 05/05/94
M3. INSULIN, REG                     SC  QID   V3. 05/03/94  INP-MED
M4. CARAFATE              1 GM       PO  QID   V4. 05/03/94
M5. ALDACTONE           25 MG       PO  BID    V5. 05/02/94  ES-ER
M6. DECADRON TAPER       3 MG       PO  TID    V6. 04/28/94  ES-ER
M7. NPH INSULIN         80 UNIT     SC  BID    V7. 04/26/94  BIMA
M8. MVI                     1       PO  QD     V8. 04/25/94  BIMA
                                               (more)
A ALLERGIES        F FUTURE APPTS    +H HEALTH MAINT.     L LAB LOOKUP
M MEDICATIONS      +N NOTES           P PROBLEMS          S VITAL SIGNS
+T TO-DO LIST      V VISIT DISPLAY    -X EXTRA FUNCTIONS
CHOICE: _
```

Figure 4-1. Patient Summary Screen from BICS Ambulatory Record

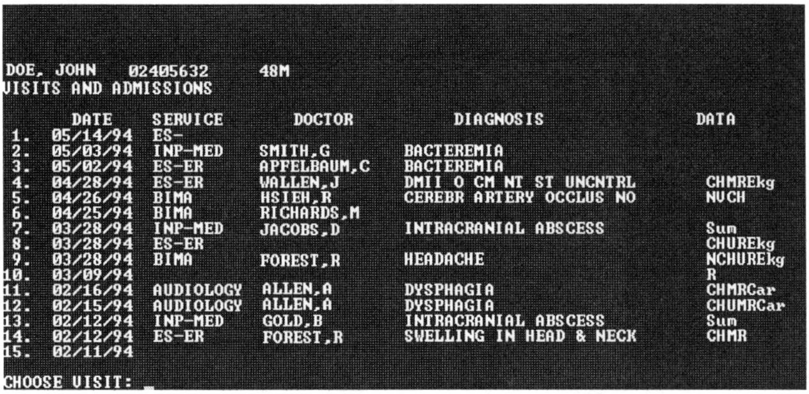

```
DOE, JOHN      02405632      48M
VISITS AND ADMISSIONS

      DATE       SERVICE       DOCTOR          DIAGNOSIS                  DATA
 1.  05/14/94   ES-
 2.  05/03/94   INP-MED     SMITH,G         BACTEREMIA
 3.  05/02/94   ES-ER       APFELBAUM,C     BACTEREMIA
 4.  04/28/94   ES-ER       WALLEN,J        DMII O CM NT ST UNCNTRL      CHMREkg
 5.  04/26/94   BIMA        HSIEH,R         CEREBR ARTERY OCCLUS NO      NUCH
 6.  04/25/94   BIMA        RICHARDS,M
 7.  03/28/94   INP-MED     JACOBS,D        INTRACRANIAL ABSCESS         Sum
 8.  03/28/94   ES-ER                                                    CHUREkg
 9.  03/28/94   BIMA        FOREST,R        HEADACHE                     NCHUREkg
10.  03/09/94                                                            R
11.  02/16/94   AUDIOLOGY   ALLEN,A         DYSPHAGIA                    CHMRCar
12.  02/15/94   AUDIOLOGY   ALLEN,A         DYSPHAGIA                    CHUMRCar
13.  02/12/94   INP-MED     GOLD,B          INTRACRANIAL ABSCESS         Sum
14.  02/12/94   ES-ER       FOREST,R        SWELLING IN HEAD & NECK      CHMR
15.  02/11/94

CHOOSE VISIT: _
```

Figure 4-2. "Day at a Glance" Screen from BICS Ambulatory Record

section collates all pertinent data and automatically fills in items that are stored elsewhere in BICS such as cholesterol and Pap smear results. Each physician's or nurse's daily schedule is also available online and is linked to the record. Thus, a user can arrive at work in the morning, see which patients are scheduled for the day, and review the records on any or all of them directly from the schedule display. Users can also enter "to do" items for any of their patients and view all to-do items each day to see what is pending in the entire practice.

Among the major incentives for data entry are value and convenience. Physicians and nurses are generally working within ambulatory records for most of the day, so the system is always at-hand for entry of a new note or a medication change. When they need to document a telephone call with a patient, the physician or nurse can type the note directly into the record, without waiting for the paper medical record to arrive.

Longer notes are entered by dictation. The transcription service sends the notes back to BICS via modem transfer; recognition software locates key fields in the transcribed note and assigns the note to the proper provider and visit. In some practices, structured entry flowsheets have been built that allow some or all of the day's notes to be entered in a rapid tabular form; this increases the speed of entering notes online and reduces the reliance on dictation.

There is a "critical mass" effect regarding the amount of data contained in the record and its value to the user. When the first practice was started on the computerized record, little pre-existing data were available in the computer for the provider's benefit. In addition, the practice had already been using a problem list and a medication list, entered by hand on a single sheet of each patient's record. When the record was first implemented, the provider had to copy these into the computer record when the patient came for their next visit. Until most patients were back for their second visit, the computer caused more extra work than it saved. When the record was introduced into the second practice, existing documentation concerning problems and medications was transcribed in advance by a medical student or secretary. Additionally, progress notes for prior visits were obtained from the transcription service and copied into the computer. In this way, the past medical history and recent progress notes were already set up for the patients in the practice, and the computerized record was a net benefit to users from the first day of operation.

Emergency Department

Several interrelated programs on BICS serve the Emergency Department (ED): the Department Log and the "Expect" Log.

The Department Log (Figure 4-3) tracks each patient who is currently in the ED, from the time the patient registers to the time of discharge from the department. The display of the log appears on most workstations in the department when the workstation is not otherwise in use, so the information it provides is always available. The log shows each patient's time of arrival, name and record number, current location in the department, chief complaint, treating physician and nurse, and status. All of these data are entered in one form or another by the department secretary, nurse, or physician.

Many of the preceding functions have been in place for many years, going back to the initial introduction of patient care computer systems at BWH. Recent developments have added further value to the log. New fields have been added to the display, showing how many laboratory tests of each type have been completed, whether the patient has a preexisting ambulatory-record file, and whether the patient is an "expected" patient (see later). Also displayed are various events that may have been entered elsewhere. These include assignment of an inpatient bed, availability of emergency blood products at the Blood Bank, Rh-

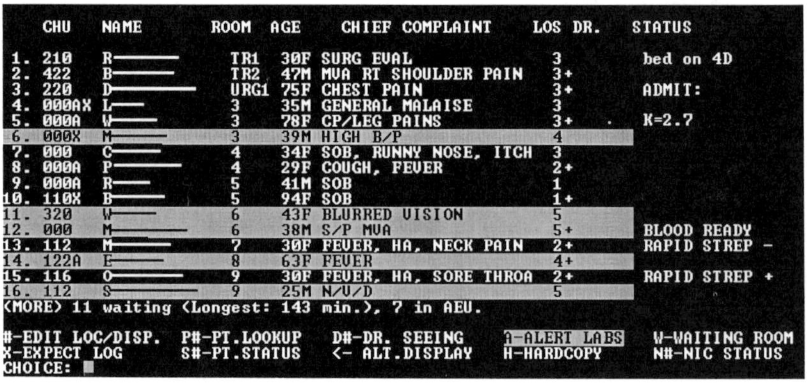

```
     CHU    NAME        ROOM  AGE    CHIEF COMPLAINT      LOS DR.   STATUS

 1.  210    R───────    TR1   30F  SURG EVAL              3        bed on 4D
 2.  422    B───────    TR2   47M  MVA RT SHOULDER PAIN   3+
 3.  220    D───────    URG1  75F  CHEST PAIN             3+       ADMIT:
 4.  000AX  L───────    3     35M  GENERAL MALAISE        3
 5.  000A   W───────    3     78F  CP/LEG PAINS           3+   .   K=2.7
 6.  000X   M───────    3     39M  HIGH B/P               4
 7.  000    C───────    4     34F  SOB, RUNNY NOSE, ITCH  3
 8.  000A   P───────    4     29F  COUGH, FEVER           2+
 9.  000A   R───────    5     41M  SOB                    1
10.  110X   B───────    5     94F  SOB                    1+
11.  320    W───────    6     43F  BLURRED VISION         5
12.  000    M───────    6     38M  S/P MVA                5+       BLOOD READY
13.  112    M───────    7     30F  FEVER, HA, NECK PAIN   2+       RAPID STREP -
14.  122A   E───────    8     63F  FEVER                  4+
15.  116    O───────    9     30F  FEVER, HA, SORE THROA  2+       RAPID STREP +
16.  112    S───────    9     25M  N/U/D                  5
<MORE> 11 waiting <Longest: 143 min.>, 7 in AEU.

#-EDIT LOC/DISP.    P#-PT.LOOKUP    D#-DR. SEEING    A-ALERT LABS    W-WAITING ROOM
X-EXPECT LOG        S#-PT.STATUS    <- ALT.DISPLAY   H-HARDCOPY      N#-NIC STATUS
CHOICE: █
```

Figure 4-3. Emergency Department Log from BICS

factor status, results of rapid strep testing, drug-resistant bacteria history, and several others.

The automated Department Log has become a valuable organizational tool for the department. A physician or nurse can look up patient information simply by choosing the patient from the listing on the log, an easier process than looking up the patient separately. Highlights and boldface entries alert the user to important facts, such as the presence of alert labs or an excessive length of stay in the department. Entries can be made on patients via the log for medical records or for quality-assurance purposes. There is an incentive to enter these data because it remains available permanently once entered, and can be used to help communicate information or to save data for later analysis.

The attending physician and charge nurse often travel rapidly from room to room, observing patient status and making interventions and notes. To support this typical work pattern, users can request a printout of the log display, use the printout to record scratch notes, and then enter any necessary information into the system. (This and other "walk-around" functions are logical targets for the application of hand-held computers in the future.)

The Expect Log (Figure 4-4) lists all patients who are expected (i.e., their physician called in advance to notify the BWH). Physicians at an outside office (including at the BWH's primary HMO and other remote locations) can also enter patients directly online, an access tool that eliminates the need for telephone calls between busy providers. In practice, the BWH is notified of about 40 percent of referred patients in this way. When the expect note is written, the system forwards a request to medical records to pull the patient's chart and deliver it to the ED. The expect note is printed at the nursing station and is displayed whenever a user looks up information concerning the patient.

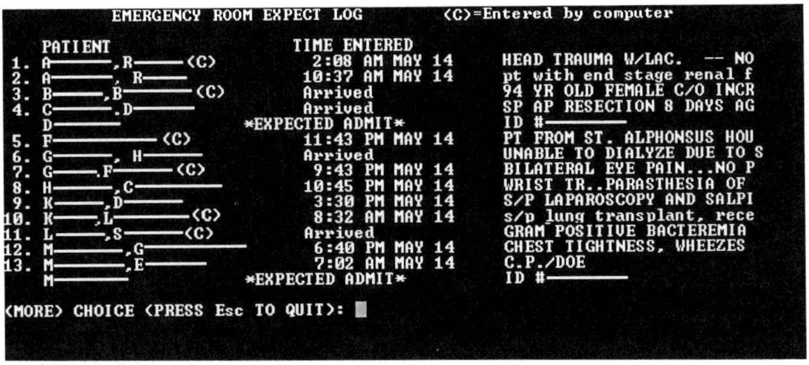

Figure 4-4. Emergency Department Expect Log from BICS

Other applications supporting the ED carry information from the log directly to the follow-up system, which keeps track of abnormal laboratory and culture results that may be filed after the patient is discharged. This supports the follow-up process by providing extra information to the reviewer such as diagnosis, previous laboratory results, and available telephone numbers should the reviewer wish to contact the patient. The reviewer can use the computer to print out a letter to the patient or to place a note in the patient's medical record. The follow-up system also takes care of required administrative functions such as mandatory public-health reporting of certain diseases, without human intervention.

Physician Order Entry

All orders for medical, surgical, orthopedic, and gynecologic patients on acute care and intensive care units at BWH are currently entered through BICS.(78,113,114) Over 90 percent are entered by physicians; the rest are entered by nurses in response to voice orders. In all, 12,000-14,000 orders are entered each day.

Physicians can enter orders on any patient from any workstation, including remote workstations in offices and homes if the user has the appropriate security arrangements. This universal access saves residents from having to walk back to each unit after rounds to write orders in the chart, and eliminates the frustration of trying to write orders when the chart is not on the unit. This universal access also greatly reduces the number of verbal orders, because the primary reason (i.e., physician is too far away to write the order) is eliminated.

Like other BICS applications, order entry uses a windowed interface. Screens are specially designed for each type of order–medications, laboratory tests, and so on. These *assisted mode* screens help the user with prompts for required fields and useful related information. For example, when a physician is ordering furosemide, the latest potassium lab result is displayed (Figure 4-5); when blood

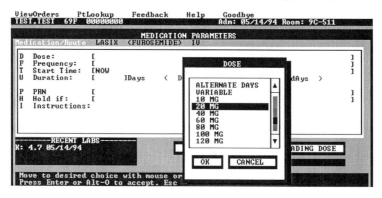

Figure 4-5. Assisted Mode Order Entry Screen from BICS (Including Latest Potassium Display with Order for Furosemide)

products are being ordered, the screen displays any transfusion restrictions for the patient and notifies the user whether the Blood Bank has a usable crossmatch specimen. The screen design also tries to make entering straightforward orders as quick as possible by providing acceptable default values, while allowing for complex orders with special instructions and fields. Default doses and frequencies for medications are based on recommendations from the BWH Pharmacy and Therapeutics Committee. Where there are no recommendations, defaults are taken from a survey of 300,000 medication orders written at the hospital over a 6-month period.

Though the assisted mode screens give the most information to the ordering physician, other screens favor speed and convenience of ordering. *Quick mode* ordering allows a user to simply type in an order, as it might be written by hand. A text parser understands most typed orders for medications, laboratory tests, and blood products, including complex doses and time schedules (Figure 4-6). The parser asks the user to confirm its interpretation of the order, and then processes the typed string of characters as it would any assisted mode order. Although quick mode is faster, only 7 percent of orders are written in this way, possibly because beginning users learn to use the assisted screens first and become comfortable with them.

Order sets and templates are used when a situation calls for a group of orders that are often ordered together. For example, when a patient is admitted, orders are needed in a variety of areas: diagnosis and condition, vital-signs checks and intravenous fluids, allergies and diets, X-rays and laboratory tests. The admission template (Figure 4-7) places all of these ordering options on one screen; the physician enters or checks parameters for each order. Order sets and templates can be used to help organize and guide the orders for any number of specific situations; one supports orders given in the intensive care unit, another facilitates orders after total-knee-replacement surgery. Physicians may create and use their own personal order sets at any time, but these sets remain private; only officially approved departmental order sets are available to all. Approximately 25 percent of all orders entered come from order sets and templates.

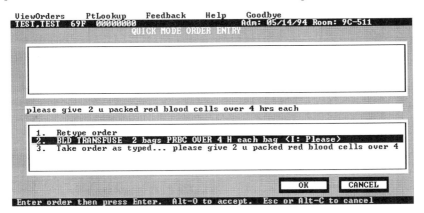

Figure 4-6. Quick Mode Order Entry Screen from BICS

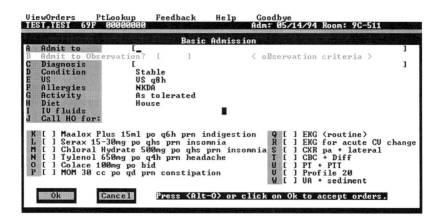

```
ViewOrders    PtLookup    Feedback    Help    Goodbye
TEST,TEST   69F  00000000                  Adm: 05/14/94  Room: 9C-511
                          Basic Admission
A  Admit to            [_                                               ]
B  Admit to Observation?  [    ]          < oBservation criteria >
C  Diagnosis           [                                               ]
D  Condition           Stable
E  US                  US q8h
F  Allergies           NKDA
G  Activity            As tolerated
H  Diet                House
I  IV fluids                             ▮
J  Call HO for:

K  [ ] Maalox Plus 15ml po q6h prn indigestion    Q  [ ] EKG (routine)
L  [ ] Serax 15-30mg po qhs prn insomnia          R  [ ] EKG for acute CV change
M  [ ] Chloral Hydrate 500mg po qhs prn insomnia  S  [ ] CXR pa + lateral
N  [ ] Tylenol 650mg po q4h prn headache          T  [ ] CBC + Diff
O  [ ] Colace 100mg po bid                         U  [ ] PT + PTT
P  [ ] MOM 30 cc po qd prn constipation            V  [ ] Profile 20
                                                    W  [ ] UA + sediment

     Ok          Cancel      Press <Alt-O> or click on Ok to accept orders.
```

Figure 4-7. Admission Template Screen from Order Entry in BICS

Certain clinical scenarios call for a different sort of information flow than is normally provided for in order entry software. BICS order entry provides special modes of display and input to allow managing these situations easily. For example, at BWH many orthopedic surgery patients are placed on warfarin postoperatively, to prevent the formation of blood clots. The daily dosage of this drug is dependent upon the results of a laboratory test, the normalized prothrombin time (PT). The physician covering this service usually reviews the results for all of the patients on the service each evening, and specifies the appropriate daily dose for each. Rather than require the physician to view results and then enter the order for each patient separately, BICS provides a spreadsheet showing all patients on the service, with the week's PT results displayed for each. The physician can select a patient, enter a dose of warfarin, then immediately move to the next patient, covering 20 or more patients in a few minutes. Other programs handle the special ordering requirements of transferred patients, patients moving through the recovery room, patients needing pre-admission orders, and complex medication orders such as sliding scales.

Computer order entry offers many opportunities to improve the organization and communication of orders. As soon as an order is electronically signed, monitors at the nursing station notify the nurse that there are pending orders designating stat and one-time orders as such (BICS does not yet support nursing due lists). At the same time, the order is being forwarded to ancillary services: medication orders to the nearest pharmacy station, X-ray orders printed or displayed in radiology. If approval is needed for an urgent radiology study, the request can be forwarded directly to the radiologist.

Because all orders entered into BICS are in a database, they can be called up and grouped for display in a number of different ways. A user can ask to view only the orders of one type, only active orders, expanded order information, and more. All of the orders are legible and the name of the entering physician is readable. The time when each order was written and when it was acknowledged by the nurse are both recorded for use in process management.

One of the most important justifications for physician order entry is the potential for improving care. Orders directly reflect the physician's care plan for the patient; the best time to influence the physician's care plan is at the time the orders are being written. In BICS, default medication doses and frequencies established by the hospital pharmacy remind the physician of standard practice. These recommendations can be easily overridden if the physician wishes to use a different dose. The display of related laboratory tests on medication-order screens helps the physician head off potential complications. The system can give warnings if the patient is allergic to an ordered medication, if the medication conflicts or interacts with other orders, if a new laboratory result affects a prior order, or for any other conditions that the computer can detect based on the information it has captured. A recent study at BWH showed that a computer armed with order entry and event-detection logic can prevent 20 percent or more of adverse in-hospital events.(115)

Order entry can also help in promoting hospital policies and cost-conscious care. BICS displays the charges to be assessed for laboratory tests and radiology procedures as shown in Figure 4-8. A study is currently underway to determine the effect of this display on the cost of inpatient care. Previous work has demonstrated that substantial cost savings can be achieved.(116) Advisory messages appear when an inexpensive drug is available that may give equal benefit to an ordered expensive drug, or when an ordered procedure or test has already been done very recently.

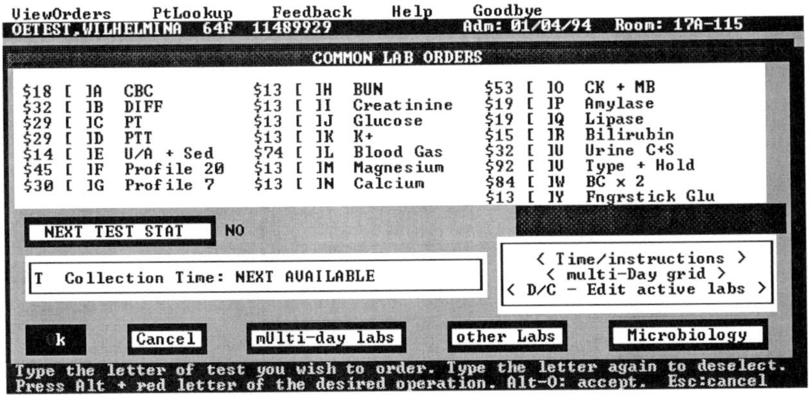

```
ViewOrders    PtLookup    Feedback    Help    Goodbye
OETEST,WILHELMINA  64F   11489929              Adm: 01/04/94   Room: 17A-115
                            COMMON LAB ORDERS
$18 [ ]A  CBC          $13 [ ]H  BUN          $53 [ ]O  CK + MB
$32 [ ]B  DIFF         $13 [ ]I  Creatinine   $19 [ ]P  Amylase
$29 [ ]C  PT           $13 [ ]J  Glucose      $19 [ ]Q  Lipase
$29 [ ]D  PTT          $13 [ ]K  K+           $15 [ ]R  Bilirubin
$14 [ ]E  U/A + Sed    $74 [ ]L  Blood Gas    $32 [ ]U  Urine C+S
$45 [ ]F  Profile 20   $13 [ ]M  Magnesium    $92 [ ]U  Type + Hold
$30 [ ]G  Profile 7    $13 [ ]N  Calcium      $84 [ ]W  BC x 2
                                              $13 [ ]Y  Fngrstick Glu

 NEXT TEST STAT    NO

 T   Collection Time: NEXT AVAILABLE           < Time/instructions >
                                                 < multi-Day grid >
                                               < D/C - Edit active labs >

     k      Cancel    mUlti-day labs    other Labs    Microbiology
Type the letter of test you wish to order. Type the letter again to deselect.
Press Alt + red letter of the desired operation. Alt-O: accept.  Esc:cancel
```

Figure 4-8. Order Screen from BICS Including Display of Patient Charges

Physicians throughout the hospital use the order entry system on BICS for their work. Efforts to implement physician order entry have at times met with substantial physician resistance.(67,117) The developers of BICS combined many different approaches to help ensure that there would be substantial incentives for physicians to enter orders. The combination of quick mode entry, order sets, and templates keeps any additional time to a minimum. Despite this, scribbling is still faster, especially when the patient is nearby. Initial results of an internal study suggest that order entry adds 15 minutes to a typical intern's 12-hour day.(118) Not all orders take longer; admission orders take substantially less time. BICS developers are now using the results of this analysis to further streamline those orders that take longer than necessary to enter.

Despite the small amount of additional time for physicians, order entry is well received. Value-added features provide much of the incentive. Related laboratory tests, calculations for total parenteral nutrition, easy access from multiple locations, automatic flow of orders to the appropriate locations, suggested doses and parameters, reminders and alerts, and order sets all combine to make the system worthwhile to the physicians. A sense of ownership of the system promotes user satisfaction as well, perhaps far more than any design feature. Suggestions for improvement are solicited from the physicians on an ongoing basis, and a development team meets weekly to review these suggestions and act on them as appropriate.

References

1. Cort R, Crawford AG. Tackling the technology. *In* Abrami PF, Johnson JE (eds). Bringing Computers to the Hospital Bedside. New York: Springer Publishing Company, 1990;16-27.
2. Dick RS, Steen EB. The Computer-Based Patient Record: An Essential Technology for Health Care. Washington, DC: National Academy Press, 1991.
3. Zielstorff RD, Hudgings CF, Grobe SF. Next-Generation Nursing Information Systems. Essential Characteristics for Professional Practice.Washington, DC: American Nurses Association, 1993.
4. Shneiderman, B. Response time and display rate in human performance with computers. Computing Surveys 1984;16:265-285.
5. Zielstorff RD, McHugh ML, Clinton J. Computer Design Criteria For Systems That Support the Nursing Process. Kansas City, MI: American Nurses' Association, 1988.
6. Kolodner RM. Functional workstation requirements: clinical perspectives. International Journal of Biomedical Computing 1994;34(1-4):116-121.
7. Childs BW. Four keys for creating the physician-IS interface. Healthcare Informatics 1993;August:4.

8. Brown A, MacDonald R. Types of point-of-care clinical computing systems and their role in different clinical environments. Proceedings of the 1991 Annual HIMSS Conference, Chicago, IL: American Hospital Association 1991;179-189.
9. Halford G, Burkes M, Pryor TA. Measuring the impact of bedside terminals. Nursing Management 1989;20:41-45.
10. Drazen E. How to select the right bedside system. Straight talk on bedside terminals. Presentation at the "User-to-User Straight Talk on Bedside Terminals" Conference, United Communications, Washington, DC, April 16, 1993.
11. Sherwood P, Poleto MC. Integrating nursing documentation, acuity classification, and cost accounting systems. Proceedings of the 1993 Annual HIMSS Conference, Chicago, IL: American Hospital Association, 1993;2:164-184.
12. Grewal R, Arcus J, Bowen J, et al. Bedside computerization of the ICU. Design Issues: Benefits of computerization versus ease of pen & paper. Proceedings of the 15th Annual SCAMC. McGraw-Hill, Inc., 1992;793-797.
13. McDonald CJ, Tierney WM, Martin DK, et al. The Regenstreif medical record 1991: a campus-wide system. Proceedings of the 15th Annual SCAMC. McGraw-Hill, Inc., 1992;925-928.
14. Safran C, Rury C, Rind D et al. Outpatient medical records for a teaching hospital. Beginning the physician-computer dialogue. Proceedings of the 15th Annual SCAMC. McGraw-Hill, Inc., 1992;114-118.
15. Anonymous. The Evolution of a Community Network. Community Medical Network Society, November 1993.
16. Teach RI, Shortliffe E. Analysis of physician attitudes regarding computer-based clinical consultation systems. Computers in Biomedical Research 1981;14:542-558.
17. Bria WF, Rydell RL. The Physician-Computer Connection. A Practical Guide to Physician Involvement in Hospital Information Systems. Chicago, IL: American Hospital Association, 1992.
18. Beck JR, Barnett GO, Clayton PD, et al. Terminals and workstations for computer-based records. In Ball MJ, Collen MF (eds). Aspects of the Computer-Based Patient Record. New York: Springer Verlag, 1992;99-101.
19. Michael PA. Physician-directed software design: the role of utilization statistics and user input in enhancing HELP results review capabilities. Proceedings of the 17th Annual SCAMC. McGraw-Hill, Inc., 1994;107-111.
20. Teich JM, Hurley JF, Beckley RF et al. Design of an easy-to-use physician order entry system with support for nursing and ancillary departments. Proceedings of the 16th Annual SCAMC. McGraw-Hill, Inc., 1993;99-103.

21. Sidelli RV, Johnson SB, Clayton PD. Full-text document storage and retrieval in a clinical information system. Topics in Health Information Management 1993;13:36-50.
22. Bleich HW, Beckley RF, Horowitz GL, et al. Clinical computing in a teaching hospital. New England Journal of Medicine 1985;312:756-764.
23. Personal communication with COL George Underwood, MD, CHCS Physician Project Officer, Tripler Army Medical Center, Honolulu, HI.
24. McDonald CJ, Tierney WM, Overhage JM, et al. The Regenstreif Medical Record System: 20 years of experience in hospitals, clinics, and neighborhood health centers. MD Computing 1992;9:206-217.
25. Henke J, Whiting-O'Keefe QE, Whiting A, et al. STOR: From pilot project to medical center implementation. Proceedings of the 12th Annual SCAMC. IEEE Publishers, 1988;733-737.
26. McCallie D, Margulies D, Kohane I, et al. The Children's Hospital clinician's workstation. Proceedings of the 14th Annual SCAMC. McGraw-Hill, Inc., 1990;755-759.
27. Teich JM, Geisler MA, Cimerman DE, et al. Design considerations in the BWH ambulatory medical record: features for maximum acceptance by clinicians. Proceedings of the 14th Annual SCAMC. McGraw-Hill, Inc., 1990;735-739.
28. Stead WM, Pryor DB, Smith PK, et al. Hospital information systems: a clinician's expectations. In Bakker AR, Ball MJ, Scherrer JR, et al. eds. Towards New Hospital Information Systems. Amsterdam:Elsevier (North-Holland), 1988;329-335.
29. Rowberg AH, Price TD. The need and user requirements for integrating images with radiology reports. Proceedings of the 15th Annual SCAMC. McGraw-Hill, Inc., 1992;163-167.
30. London JW, Morton DE. The integration of text, graphics, and radiographic images on X-terminal clinical workstations. Proceedings of MEDINFO 92. Amsterdam:Elsevier (North-Holland), 1992;41-46.
31. Bradshaw KE, Gardner RM, Clemmer TP, et al. Physician decision-making–evaluation of data used in a computerized ICU. International Journal of Clinical Monitoring and Computing 1984;1:81-91.
32. Tang PC, Annevelink J, Fafchamps D, et al. Physicians' workstations: integrated information management for clinicians. Proceedings of the 15th Annual SCAMC. McGraw-Hill, Inc., 1992;569-573.
33. Tate KE, Gardner RM. Computers, quality, and the clinical laboratory. Proceedings of the 17th Annual SCAMC. McGraw-Hill, Inc., 1994;193-197.
34. Hammond WE. TMR–A profile of an electronic medical record. Proceedings of MEDINFO 92. Amsterdam:Elsevier (North-Holland), 1992;730-736.

35. Hammond W, Stead WW. Adopting TMR for physician/nurse use. Proceedings of the 15th Annual SCAMC. McGraw-Hill, Inc., 1992;833-837.
36. Composite Health Care System Program Office, Medical Functional Information Management, U.S. Department of Defense, Falls Church, VA.
37. Safran C, Rury CD, Lightfoot J, et al. ClinQuery: a program for interactive searching of clinical data. Proceedings of the 13th Annual SCAMC. IEEE Publishers, 1989;414-418.
38. Hammond WE, Straube MJ, Blunden PB, et al. Query: the language of databases. Proceedings of the 13th Annual SCAMC. IEEE Publishers, 1989;419-423.
39. Osheroff JA, Forsythe DE, Buchanan BG, et al. Physicians' information needs: analysis of questions posed during clinical teaching. Annals of Internal Medicine 1991;114:576-581.
40. Horowitz GL, Bleich HL. PaperChase: a computer program to search the medical literature. New England Journal of Medicine 1981;305:924-930.
41. Singer J, Sacks HS, Lucente F, et al. Physician attitudes toward applications of computer database systems. Journal of the American Medical Association. 1983;249:1610-1614.
42. Sandness JG. Use of online databases by practicing physicians. Proceedings of the 13th Annual SCAMC. IEEE Publishers, 1989;456-461.
43. Gorman P. Does the medical literature contain the evidence to answer the questions of primary care physicians? Preliminary findings of a study. Proceedings of the 17th Annual SCAMC. McGraw-Hill, Inc., 1994;571-575.
44. Humphreys BL, Lindberg DAB. The Unified Medical Language System Project: a distributed experiment in improving access to biomedical information. Proceedings of MEDINFO 92. Amsterdam:Elsevier (North-Holland), 1992;1496-1499.
45. Cimino JJ, Johnson SB, Aguirre A, et al. The Medline button. Proceedings of the 16th Annual SCAMC. McGraw-Hill, Inc., 1993;81-85.
46. Miller RA, Gieszcykiewicz FM, Vries JK, et al. CHARTLINE: providing bibliographic references relevant to patient charts using the UMLS Metathesaurus Knowledge Sources. Proceedings of the 16th Annual SCAMC. McGraw-Hill, Inc., 1993;86-90.
47. Tuttle MS, Sheretz DD, Fagan LM, et al. Toward an interim standard for patient-centered knowledge access. Proceedings of the 17th Annual SCAMC. McGraw-Hill, Inc., 1994;564-568.
48. Tuttle MS, Sheretz DD, Fagan LM, et al. Toward a patient-centered knowledge-server standard for CPRs. Proceedings of the Annual HIMSS Conference, Chicago, IL: Health Information Management System Society, 1994;Vol 2:115-128.
49. Safran C, Hermann F, Rind D, et al. Computer-based support for clinical decision making. M.D. Computing 1990;7:319-322.

50. Bikson TK, Gutek BA, Mankin DA. Implementing Computerized Procedures in Office Settings. Influences and Outcomes. R-3077-NSF/IRIS. Santa Monica, CA: The RAND Corporation, 1987.

51. Lurie N, Rank B, Parenti C, et al. How do house officers spend their nights? A time study of internal medicine house staff on call. New England Journal of Medicine 1989;320:1673-1677.

52. Overhage JM, Tierney WM, McDonald CJ, et al. How do interns spend their days: a time-motion study of internal medicine interns. Clinical Research 1991;39:794A.

53. Lange LL. Information-seeking by nurses during beginning-of-shift activities. Proceedings of the 16th Annual SCAMC. McGraw-Hill, Inc., 1993;317-321.

54. Forsythe DE, Buchanan BG. Expanding the concept of medical information: An observational study of physicians' information needs. Computers and Biomedical Research 1992;25:181-200.

55. Fafchamps D, Young CY, Tang PC. Modelling work practices: input to the design of a physician's workstation. Proceedings of the 15th Annual SCAMC. McGraw-Hill, Inc., 1992;788-792.

56. Malbin K, Putz B, Mitchell M, et al. The process and outcome of a collaborative effort to design and implement a clinician order processing system. Proceedings of the 16th Annual SCAMC. McGraw-Hill, Inc., 1993;785-786.

57. Nowlan AW. Clinical workstations: identifying clinical requirements and understanding clinical information. International Journal of Bio-Medical Computing 1994;34(1-4):85-94.

58. Hravnak M, Stein KL, Dale B, et al. Ongoing development of the critical care information system: The collaborative approach to automating information management in an intensive care unit. Proceedings of the 16th Annual SCAMC. McGraw-Hill, Inc., 1993;3-7.

59. Connelly DP, Werth DW, Hultman BK, et al. Physician use of an NICU laboratory reporting system. Proceedings of the 15th Annual SCAMC. McGraw-Hill, Inc., 1993;8-12.

60. Rochman R. Facilitating and enhancing the role of the nurse: The nurse and the clinical workstation. In Marr PB, Axford RL, Newbold SK, eds. Nursing Informatics '91. Proceedings of the Post Conference on Health Care Information Technology: Implications for Change. Springer Verlag 1991;105-111.

61. Ball MJ, Silva JS, Douglas JV et al. The health care professional workstation. Proceedings of a working conference sponsored by the International Medical Information Association. International Journal of Bio-Medical Computing 1994;34(1-4):1-416.

62. Kolodner RM. Functional workstation requirements: clinical perspectives. International Journal of Bio-Medical Computing 1994;34:115-121.

63. Chignell MH, Hancock PA, Loewenthal A. An introduction to intelligent interfaces 1-22, *In* Hancock PA, Chignell MH. (eds). Intelligent interfaces. Theory, research, and design. Amsterdam: North-Holland, 1989:1-22.
64. Safran C. Defining clinical workstation. International Journal of Bio-Medical Computing 1994;34(1-4):261-265.
65. Clayton PD, Pulver GE, Hill CL. Physician use of computers: is age or value the predominant factor? Proceedings of the 17th Annual Symposium on Computer Applications in Medical Care. McGraw-Hill, Inc., 1994:301-305.
66. Turley JP, Connelly DP. The relationship between nursing and medical cultures: Implications for the design and implementation of a clinician's workstation.Proceedings of the 17th Annual SCAMC. McGraw-Hill, Inc., 1994:233-237.
67. Massaro TA. Introducing physician order entry at a major academic medical center. II. Impact on medical education. Academic Medicine 1993;68:25-30.
68. Zibrack JD, Roberts MS, Nelick-Cohen L, et al. Creating an environment conducive to physician participation in a hospital information system. Proceedings of the 14th Annual SCAMC. IEEE Publishers, 1990;779-783.
69. O'Dell DV, Tape TG, Campbell JR. Increasing physician acceptance and use of the computerized ambulatory record. Proceedings of the 15th Annual SCAMC. McGraw-Hill, Inc. 1992;848-852.
70. Ischar R, Aydin CE. Predicting effective use of hospital computer systems. Proceedings of the 12th Annual SCAMC. IEEE Publishers, 1988;862-868.
71. Staggers N. Human factors. The missing element in computer technology. Computers in Nursing 1991;9:47-49.
72. Work Group on Computerization of Patient Records. Toward a National Health Information Infrastructure. Report to the Secretary of the U.S. Department of Health and Human Services, April 1993.
73. Government Accounting Office. Medical ADP Systems. Automated Records Hold Promise to Improve Patient Care. GAO/IMTEC-91-5. Washington, DC, 1991.
74. Witte VR, Matthews P. Managing change through nursing informatics. Proceedings of the 1992 Annual HIMSS Conference, Chicago, IL: American Hospital Association, 1992;93-100.
75. Boyer A, Levine HS. Automation of clinical documentation–an in-depth assessment from the care giver's perspective. Proceedings of the 1993 Annual HIMSS Conference, Chicago, IL: Health Information Management System Society, 1993;1:15-25.
76. Andreshak JC, Lumelsky S, Chang IF, et al. Medication charting via computer gesture recognition. Proceedings of the 14th Annual SCAMC. IEEE Publishers, 1990;865-869.
77. Chang MM. Clinician-entered computerized psychiatric triage records. Hospital and Community Psychiatry 1987;38:652-656.
78. Teich JM, Hurley JF, Beckley RF, et al. Design of an easy-to-use physician order entry system with support for nursing and ancillary

departments. Proceedings of the 16th Annual SCAMC. McGraw-Hill, Inc., 1992;99-103.

79. Pryor A. Current state of computer-based patient records. 67-82. In Ball M, Collen M (eds.) Aspects of the Computer-Based Patient Record. Springer Verlag 1992.

80. Sittig DF, Stead WM. Computer-based physician order entry: the state of the art. Journal of the American Medical Informatics Association 1994;1:108-123.

81. Gibbons PS, Anderson AJ, Drossel LM, et al. Coordinated delivery of clinical care: The "re-integration" of the medical group practice. Proceedings of the 16th Annual SCAMC. McGraw-Hill, Inc., 1993;64-68.

82. Overhage JM, Tierney WM, Martin JM, et al. Computer-assisted order entry: Impact on intern time. Clinical Research 1991;39:794A.

83. Potolicchio S, Hylton J, Broering NC, et al. Enhancing clinical investigation in neurology with a patient information system. Proceedings of the 12th Annual SCAMC. IEEE Publishers, 1988;688-692.

84. Siders AM, Peterson M. Increasing patient satisfaction and nursing productivity through implementation of an automated nursing discharge summary. Proceedings of the 15th Annual SCAMC. McGraw-Hill, Inc., 1992;136-140.

85. Grewal R, Arcus J, Bowen J, et al. Design and development of an automated nursing note. Proceedings of the Seventh World Congress on Medical Informatics (MEDINFO 92). Amsterdam:North-Holland, 1992;1054-1058.

86. Campbell KE, Wieckert K, Fagan LM, et al. A computer-based tool for generation of progress notes. Proceedings of the 17th Annual SCAMC. McGraw-Hill, Inc., 1994;284-288.

87. Campbell JR. Content and organization of the computerized ambulatory record. Proceedings of the 17th Annual SCAMC. McGraw-Hill, Inc., 1994;863.

88. Cimino JJ, Barnett GO. The physician's workstation: recording a physical examination using a controlled vocabulary. Proceedings of the 11th SCAMC. IEEE Publishers, 1987;287-291.

89. Clark AS, Shea S. Developing a controlled vocabulary for the Columbia-Presbyterian Medical Center outpatient clinical information system. Proceedings of the 14th Annual SCAMC. IEEE Publishers, 1990;205-209.

90. Payne TS, Martin DR. How useful is the UMLS Metathesaurus in developing a controlled vocabulary for an automated problem list? Proceedings of the 17th Annual SCAMC. McGraw-Hill, Inc., 1994;705-709.

91. Kuperman. Issues in the creation of on-line problem lists. Panel Presentation at Spring AMIA Meeting, 1993.

92. Huff SM, Pryor TA, Tebbs RD. Pick from thousands. A collaborative processing model for coded data entry. Proceedings of the 15th Annual SCAMC. McGraw-Hill, Inc., 1992;104-108.
93. Safran C, Rury C, Rind D, et al. A computer-based outpatient medical record for a teaching hospital. M.D. Computing 1991;8:291-299.
94. Dewey JB, Manning P, Brandt S. Acceptance of direct physician access to a computer-based patient record in a managed care setting. Proceedings of the 17th Annual SCAMC. McGraw-Hill, Inc., 1994;79-83.
95. Rind DM, Safran C. Real and imagined barriers to an electronic medical record. Proceedings of the 17th Annual SCAMC. McGraw-Hill Inc., 1994;74-78.
96. Laughlin ML. User interfaces: where the rubber meets the road. Computers in Healthcare 1993;February:16-22.
97. Murchie CJ, Kenny GNC. Comparison of keyboard, light pen, and voice recognition as methods of data input. International Journal of Clinical Monitoring and Computing 1988;5:243-246.
98. Trofino J. Voice-recognition technology applied to nursing documentation. Healthcare Information Management 1993;7:41-45.
99. Tang P, Patel VL. Major issues in user interface design for health professional workstations: summary and recommendations. International Journal of Bio-Medical Computing 1994;34(1-4):139-148.
100. Collinson PO, Jones RG, Howes M, et al. Of mice and men–data capture in the clinical environment. International Journal of Clinical Monitoring and Computing 1989;6:217-222.
101. Levy AH, Lawrence DP. Data acquisition for the computer-based patient record. 125-139 In Ball MJ, Collen MF (eds). Aspects of the Computer-Based Patient Record. New York: Springer Verlag, 1992.
102. Hughes S. Information systems that support patient care delivery and nursing practice. Proceedings of the 1993 Annual HIMSS Conference, Chicago, IL: Health Information Management System Society, 1993;3: 181-190.
103. Roberts MS, Zibrack JD, Siders A, et al. The development of an on-line, partially automated discharge summary and core clinical database in an existing hospital information system. Proceedings of the 13th Annual SCAMC. IEEE Publishers, 1989;649-653.
104. Petersen P. Computerized hospital information systems: a tool in quality. Presentation at the 1991 HIMSS Annual Conference, February 11-14, 1991, San Francisco.
105. Karcz A, Holbrook J, Auerbach BS, et al. Preventability of malpractice claims in emergency medicine: A closed claims study. Annals of Emergency Medicine 1990;19:865-873.
106. Zander K. Nursing case management: strategic management of cost and quality outcomes. Journal of Nursing Administration 1988;18:23-30.
107. Coffey RJ, Richards JS, Remmert CS, et al. An introduction to critical paths. Quality Management in Health Care 1992;1:45-54.

108. Ashworth GB, Aubrey C. Collaborative care documentation by exception system. Proceedings of the 16th Annual SCAMC. McGraw-Hill, Inc., 1992;109-113.
109. Burke LJ, Murphy J. Charting by Exception. A Cost-Effective, Quality Approach. Media, PA: Harwal Publishing Company, 1988.
110. Barrett MJ. Case management a must to survive managed care. Computers in Healthcare 1993;June:22-25.
111. Lumsdon K, Hagland M. Mapping care. Hospitals and Health Networks, 1993;67(19):34-40.
112. Glaser JP, Beckley RF, Roberts P, et al. A very large PC LAN as the basis for a hospital information system. Journal of Medical Systems 1991;15:133-137.
113. Teich JM, Spurr CM, Flammini SJ, et al. Response to a trial of physician-based inpatient order entry. Proceedings of the 17th Annual SCAMC, McGraw-Hill, Inc., 1994;316-320.
114. Spurr C, Glaser JP, Teich J, et al. Implementation of provider clinical order entry: One hospital's experience. Proceedings of the 1994 Annual HIMSS Conference, Chicago, IL: Health Information Management System Society, 1994;2:95-106.
115. Bates DW, O'Neill AC, Teich JM, et al. Identifiability and preventability of adverse events using information systems. Clinical Research 1993;41:PA526.
116. Tierney WM, Overhage JM, McDonald CJ. Physician inpatient order writing on microcomputer workstations. Journal of the American Medical Association 1993;269:379-383.
117. Massaro TA. Introducing physician order entry at a major academic medical center. I. Impact on organizational culture and behavior. Academic Medicine 1993;68:20-25.
118. Bates DW, Brigham and Women's Hospital (manuscript in preparation), 1994.

5
Developing a Patient Care Information System Strategy

Mark K. Schneider and William C. Reed

A recent survey of 400 hospital executives revealed that 80 percent were interested in employing patient care information systems in their institutions. Only 8 percent reported having such systems.(1) It can be a long and confusing road, from wanting patient care information systems to using patient care information systems. The journey can be made easier, however, by developing a patient care information system strategy.

Why a Patient Care Information System Strategy?

To varying degrees, all industries are dependent upon the ability to access information, at the time and in the form required. Recognizing this management challenge, organizations develop information systems strategies to facilitate their information management efforts.

An information system strategy is a template for managing information in a manner that is consistent with the strategies, objectives, and processes of an organization. As various dimensions of the organization change, the information systems strategy must be altered to reflect the new information needs.

Health care organizations need patient care information system strategies because of the competition for limited organizational resources. Information systems initiatives often require a substantial investment in capital and human resources. Both of these resource pools are limited in health care organizations. Additionally, these resources are being further constrained by capitation and reduced reimbursements.

Many health care organizations find it difficult to determine the appropriate allocation of these resources to information systems versus other projects. Frequently, such difficulty is exacerbated by the prolonged nature of information systems implementations. Having an information systems strategy mitigates this difficulty, enabling a health care organization to evaluate resource allocations more appropriately for both information systems and noninformation systems initiatives.

A strategy will explain the patient care information system in terms of understandable functionality. It is important for users, especially clinicians, to establish a comfort level as to what the patient care information system contains and how it will affect their clinical practice.

It is also important to define what the patient care information system is not. Many individuals and organizations are using rather nebulous terms, such as "computer-based patient record," to define their information system. In terms of patient care information system definition, both as to what it is and what it is not, it is critical that expectations for the patient care information system be clearly established and understood.

Every health care organization has its own personality. The patient care information system strategy takes this organizational personality into account and accommodates it in the strategy design. For example, inpatient environments need narrow and deep data stores that reflect brief episodes of care entailing repetitive collection of relatively few data points. In contrast, ambulatory care systems need to be supported by broad and shallow data stores. These systems must be more longitudinal in nature, collecting few iterations of many data points. The patient care information system strategy must take such nuances into account.

The strategy also forces a consideration of the infrastructure implications. Telecommunications implications in an inpatient environment are more easily defined than those in a home health environment. Providing workstations used in a primary care exam room by a physician demands a different strategic approach than those to be utilized at a nursing station by a ward clerk. At a high level, all of these cybernetic and technical characteristics are defined within the patient care information system strategy.

The patient care information system strategy can obviously play a vital role in ensuring the provision of efficient and effective information systems support for a health care organization. Although a "trial and error" approach to implementing a patient care information system may be ultimately successful, neither the time nor expense can be afforded in today's health care environment. Health care organizations facing major capital investments are looking to minimize the risk that investments do not achieve the desired results. Thus, a detailed strategy is needed to ensure the highest probability of success with the fewest resources.

What is a Patient Care Information System Strategy?

Pursuit of a patient care information system should be viewed as an ongoing journey rather than a specific destination, and the patient care information system strategy as a "road map" for this journey. The strategy should appropriately balance the theoretical and practical aspects of implementing a patient care information system. The theoretical aspects should focus on the reasons for installing a patient care information system and the goals and objectives to be obtained by implementing one. Yet, to gain support for the patient care information system, the strategy should be detailed enough to be understood and supported by all. Several approaches can be used in developing a strategy, but a good comprehensive patient care information strategy will have the following:

- Conceptual overview. The theoretical description of the patient care information system.
- Functional strategy. A definition of the relationship between health care activity, information needs, and information support.
- Technical strategy. The definition of the infrastructure required to support the patient care information system.
- Acquisition strategy. An explanation of the criteria to consider during the acquisition of both the functional and infrastructural components of the patient care information system.
- Migration strategy. An outline of the approach to implement the patient care information system.
- Operational and maintenance strategy. A depiction of the steps necessary to run and continually enhance the patient care information system. This may include a discrete organizational strategy.
- Implications. The nuances to be considered relative to having a patient care information system.

Conceptual Overview

The conceptual overview begins with a vision statement. The vision statement establishes the theoretical framework for the patient care information system. In very high-level terms, the vision statement explains the intent of the patient care information system.

The conceptual overview sets forth the principles that govern the patient care information system. These principles can be either relatively theoretical or very precise. They can help link institutional objectives with system direction. The principles are also used to describe both what the patient care information system is, and what it is not. Additionally, they can help to build consensus and commitment to the patient care information system.

Assumptions also are usually found in the conceptual overview. They are used to assist in describing the organizational model and the environment in which the patient care information system will function. Assumptions that may be problematic for implementation or operation of the patient care information system should be highlighted here and then further addressed in the implications section.

Functional Strategy

The functional strategy contains a description of the application portfolio required for the patient care information system or those functions that must integrate with the patient care information system. The functional strategy is developed by first identifying the generic clinical functions of the organization. Next, specific clinical functions are clustered in categories.

A model is then constructed that depicts the interrelationships among the various application areas of the patient care information system. Additionally, each application area is evaluated relative to its current level of information systems support (i.e., not automated, moderately supported, or well supported). Figure 5-1 is an example of such a model.

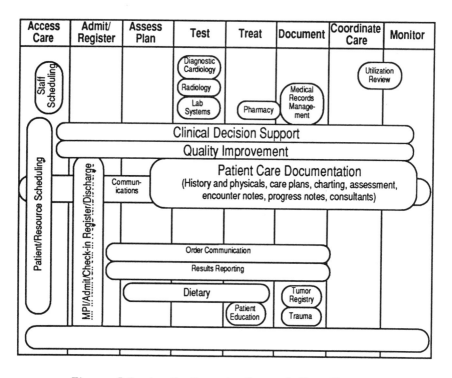

Figure 5-1. Applications to Support Key Processes

Another aspect of the functional strategy is to define the operational prerequisites that allow the patient care information system to function appropriately. These are the operational changes that must be in place before specific patient care information system functions are implemented. For example, prior to implementing a comprehensive patient scheduling system, referral authorization rules must be defined. Often, it may be more difficult and time consuming to address the operational changes than it is to implement the technical functionality. Thus, it is important for the patient care information system strategy to define both clearly.

Finally, the functional strategy provides a view of how new and existing patient care applications can support key patient care delivery roles (see Table 5-1). Many of the traditional patient care roles can be supported through purchased solutions, while unique roles (e.g., case managers) may require development of custom environments to access applications and data efficiently.

Technical Strategy

The patient care information system technical strategy provides an overview of the technical environment in which the patient care information system must function (see Figure 5-2). It should create an environment that is conducive for use by the novice as well as the experienced user.

Table 5.1. Applications to Support Key Roles

Roles	Care Planning/Documentation	MPI, ADT Registration	Patient/Resource/Staff Scheduling
	Applications		
Quality Manager	Develop care protocols • Clinical and financial outcomes Resolve provider contestations • Patient eligibility Monitor equipment and technology usage - BY-PRODUCT Monitor patient outcomes - BY-PRODUCT • Clinical/financial outcomes • Deviations from protocols Review care protocols - FEEDS INTO EIS • Clinical/financial outcomes • Deviations from protocols Establish quality program BY-PRODUCT • Quality indicators	Resolve provider contestations • Patient eligibility Track and trend provider utilization information Link treatment to physician - BY-PRODUCT • Orders • Ordering physician • Clinical/financial outcomes • Deviations from protocols Monitor provider practice - BY-PRODUCT • Admitting/ordering/referring physicians • Patients by diagnosis • Patients by resource use • Orders	Establish utilization standards • Stalling resource use by diagnosis? • Technology/equipment usage by diagnosis? Analyze utilization trends and variances • Staffing resource use by diagnosis? • Equipment/technology usage by diagnosis? • Deviations from protocols Develop staffing standards--BY-PRODUCT • Staffing resource use by diagnosis?
Multiskilled Practitioner	Assess patient condition • History, including past medical history, previous surgeries/illnesses, problem list, medicine, allergies • Physical findings, including nursing care assessment--functional system • Psycho-social needs • Admitting diagnosis • Admitting physician • Diagnostic test results • Relevant protocols • Physician orders	Assess patient condition • Admitting diagnosis • Admitting physician Plan Discharge • Psycho-social needs • Admitting diagnosis • Physician orders Prepared discharge instructions • Psycho-social needs • Admitting diagnosis • Physician orders	Assess patient condition • Physician orders • Ancillary schedules Plan transport • Physician orders • Ancillary schedules

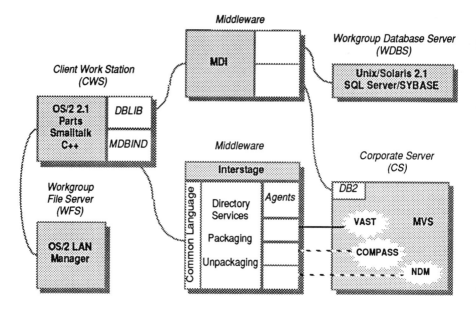

Figure 5.2. Technical Strategy

The technical characteristics of the infrastructure are of primary importance. In a patient care information system, the telecommunications aspects are extremely complex. This is especially true as the health care model embraces other components of the delivery system such as primary care sites, home health, etc.

The technical strategy should delineate specific technical standards. Some of these may be very specific (e.g., all transactions must adhere to Health Level 7 [HL7] communications protocol standards). Other standards may be somewhat less specific (e.g., all data management must be handled through a relational data manager).

Recognizing the heterogeneous nature of most patient care information systems, the technical strategy must address integration considerations. The capabilities for data, communications, and even operating platform integration must all be evaluated. Additionally, the ability to integrate different information media (e.g., voice, data, and image) should be evaluated.

Most items contained in the technical strategy should consider the following evaluation criteria:

- Ability to meet functional user requirements.
- Availability for access.
- Performance characteristics.
- Technical resource consumption.

- Business resumption considerations.
- Cost.

All aspects of the patient care information system technical strategy should subscribe to two underlying principles. First, the strategy should remain flexible. Both the evolving functional needs of users and the rapid pace of the technological change require that the technical strategy readily adapt to appropriate change. Second, the strategy should create an appropriate technical environment without excessively limiting choice. For example, the patient care information system technical strategy may state a need to utilize an industry standard programming language without specifying which language.

Acquisition Strategy

The patient care information system acquisition strategy should establish a framework for a well-defined and thorough process to acquire components that will easily integrate into the patient care information system. Such acquisitions should enhance the value of the patient care information system to clinicians while maintaining a stable operating environment. Although this portion of the strategy focuses on immediate functional needs, the long-term potential for integration should be ensured.

The presence of a patient care information system acquisition strategy does not preclude inhouse development. Rather, it establishes the ground rules for both inhouse development and external product acquisition. The strategy may encourage the use of purchased software alternatives, where available, but also recognize the need to develop, solely or cooperatively, software that is not commercially available.

When vendor products are to be utilized, the patient care information system acquisition strategy should provide direction regarding selection criteria. Such acquisition criteria should evaluate:

- To what degree does the software meet the required patient care information system functionality?
- How well does the component perform its specific function both independently and in relation to the patient care information system as a whole?
- How well can the component accommodate patient care information system growth, both in terms of volume and functionality?
- How well does the component fit technically within the patient care information system technical strategy? Although it may fit, does it introduce an unnecessary or unacceptable level of complexity?
- What has been the historical performance of the vendor? Has its offerings continued to evolve and receive adequate support?

- What is the vendor's projected stability into the future? Will the components receive the necessary support for the next 5 years?

The strategy should also offer guidance regarding the use of the health care organization as a test site for vendor products. While there are some advantages to this approach, there are also significant risks. Of primary concern in this type of environment is the clinicians' experience level with a patient care information system. Clinicians who are accustomed to interacting with a more mature patient care information system will be more likely to withstand the frustrations related to testing newly developed software. Caution should be exercised in using developmental software with clinicians who are relative novices with a patient care information system.

Prototype development is more appropriate for applications that fall in the category of "value-added" or "critical in the future" because failure of the development will not affect the institutions' ability to implement its short-term business strategy.

As a final issue, the patient care information system acquisition strategy should include appropriate references to the health care organization's system development methodology, if one is utilized.

Migration Strategy

The migration strategy describes the sequence in which clinical applications will be implemented and the process that will be utilized to facilitate successful implementation. The strategy defines discrete project tasks such as infrastructure building, new application system implementations, and organizational changes. Next, these tasks are prioritized based on clinical and strategic need. Issues of dependency and precedence are also considered in this strategy.

It is important to assess the risks associated with each task. The risk assessment considers technical risk (that the capability can be delivered), functional risk (that it will provide the expected level of support), and implementation risk (availability of a sponsor, level of process redesign required to gain benefits). These risks are viewed collectively in order to provide an overall risk associated with each task. The risk assessment will be based on an evalution of the stage of development of the technology, the information collected to develop the functional and technical plans, and the experience of other institutions that have attempted similar projects.

A good migration strategy will minimize the amount of new capital investment and provide frequent confidence-boosting deliverables. A sample migration strategy is described in Chapter 6.

Operation and Maintenance

Once the patient care information system has been implemented, its operation and maintenance become critical. The full value of the patient care information system can only be realized if it is effectively utilized and maintained. Effective utilization involves applying the patient care information system to improve the patient care delivery process in a consistent manner.

Appropriate maintenance is provided via continually improving the patient care information system to reflect changes in the health care delivery processes, enhancements to clinician interaction, and technological advancements. The operations and maintenance strategy should identify the approach to dealing with system maintenance, for example:

- New software releases will be applied when they are available and have been proven to be functionally stable.
- Requests for modifications and enhancements to the patient care information system will be addressed using a release concept. A release concept bundles multiple changes together for implementation rather than continually disrupting operations with individual changes.

Operational aspects of the strategy should clearly delineate the responsibilities of the user, the information systems managers, and the vendor.

A "concept of operations" methodology may be used to ease implementation and provide realistic user expectations. These "concepts of operations" describe the changes in operations that will occur after the system is implemented and the benefits that will be achieved. "Visualization" techniques can help show how system support for key roles will evolve.

Implications

The implications section of the patient care information system strategy addresses the management concerns related to the patient care information system. Some of these concerns may have been identified when establishing the conceptual overview, others may surface during the development of the related portions of the patient care information system strategy.

The implications may include disclosure of some subtleties related to the patient care information system.

- The value of a patient care information system is realized through the "sum of the parts" rather than individual components.
- The patient care information system often represents an "ownerless" system and thus requires concerted effort to manage.

• The patient care information system represents the sole approach to the organization's clinical automation efforts, therefore it takes precedence over grass roots effort that may have gained considerable momentum.

The Challenges

The first hurdle in developing a patient care information system plan is generating interest. While the CEO, CIO, or Director of the Medical Staff may be convinced that this is a critical blueprint for the future, the rest of the organization may see only another planning project, more committees, more meetings, more time talking, and less time doing. This indifference can be compounded by the fact that nobody has time set aside to do patient care information systems planning. The people that must help in this task are some of the busiest. If they have lots of time available, they probably should not be working on this project.

This difficulty can generally be overcome through perseverance and focus on the value of quality patient care information systems. It will be important to communicate the risks associated with bad planning (e.g., capital invested in inappropriate technologies, frustrated staff, and inappropriate measures of progress). Finally, it will be important to suggest a planning approach that is consistent with the organization's management style (more about this later).

Receiving an endorsement to develop a patient care information systems plan is only the first hurdle. Numerous other challenges are associated with planning of this type. Some of them are fairly traditional and are encountered in most systems planning efforts; some are unique to patient care information systems planning; some may be unique to the organization. There are no "silver bullets" that make these challenges go away. Adapting and customizing the process described later in this chapter will, however, certainly minimize their impact. The challenges are discussed below to assist you in anticipating, recognizing, and addressing them as they arise.

Traditional Challenges to Systems Planning

Some of the challenges associated with patient care information systems planning are common to most systems planning projects.

Executive Disinterest

Lack of executive level interest and support is probably the surest way to kill a planning initiative. Executive level interest can sometimes be absent at the very beginning due to a lack of communication or the project team's failure to link the project with business strategy and priorities. Executive interest can wane during the course of the project when it is lengthy, because of new priorities, or due to a CEO, CFO, or COO departure that leaves the project without a sponsor. Finally, the project results might not meet expectations. Expectations might not have been appropriately set at the beginning or changes not communicated during the course of the project.

The net result of any of these situations is a lack of executive-level ownership of the plan. Without ownership, it is nearly impossible to translate the plan into action. Any lack of ownership is quickly and thoroughly perceived by the rest of the organization and initiatives related to the plan are quickly discounted and devalued. Mere approval for planning is not sufficient; planning initiatives must have executive-level commitment, visible support and participation at the outset. Proactive communication during the course of the planning effort is a critical factor for success.

Translating User Needs into Systems Support

Effective systems planning begins with an understanding of needs and objectives. It then translates these into appropriate systems support functions. Several challenges are associated with completing this task effectively. The first involves focusing on the correct user needs. Dysfunctional systems result from focusing either on today's needs or on future needs without considering both. Focusing on today's needs will produce a system that is outdated before it is even built, myopically solving past problems. Focusing exclusively on the future will result in a system that can wither and die while waiting for the organization to catch up. A balance should be struck with a focus on future needs carefully leveraged with survival applications and transition plans.

Another challenge is developing systems around user roles rather than specific departments. It is much easier to design a system around the needs of a department than to solve the broader support requirement for a role or function. Designing the system around specific departments is ineffective because it renders the system obsolete when the organization changes. System design around a broader role or function protects against that obsolescence.

Another common stumbling point is the assumption by system analysts that *they* know and understand user requirements. Even when this is not an ego issue, it can frequently be a time issue. It is simply more expedient for the systems people to develop specifications or build the system based upon a few interviews because the busy physicians and nurses lack the time or motivation to participate in more in-depth analysis. The net effect of this is merely a postponement of the time investment. There will be endless revisions and rewrites later in the process. This hurdle can be addressed through process-oriented planning efforts and frequent communication, as well as CASE tools and prototyping techniques.

Finally, there are hurdles associated with translating the needs into technology solutions. The risks involve the design teams favoring extremes on the technology spectrum. Some teams, which are either risk averse or lacking vision, will favor 5-year-old familiar technology solutions. Five years is a lifetime in the information technology arena and the resulting system will be competitively disadvantaged and difficult to support in short order. At the other extreme are the design teams that tie the system's success to technology that is still in product laboratories. Though this may prove visionary in the long term, it may prove impractical in the interim.

Rapid Changes Outdate the Plan

In many businesses today (particularly in health care), we are seeing an accelerated rate of change in the way we deliver goods and services. We have lived with the constancy of change, but have yet to adapt to the new speed of change. At the same time, technology is exploding. Computer chips double in capacity and speed roughly every 2 years. This in turn drives an ever-growing multibillion dollar software industry and fuels the current revolution in telecommunications. The implication is that our information systems plan is barely printed and bound before it is labeled out-of-date. This gives the nay sayers license to ignore the plan and reminds all of the planning participants that they could have spent their time in more fruitful pursuits.

This problem can be addressed several different ways. First, it should be noted that while strategic plans generally address a 5-year horizon, *detailed* systems planning for more than 1 or 2 years hence is not very useful. As noted at the beginning of this chapter, the plan should be positioned as a road map for a longer journey, with the detail of that road map addressing only the nearer term. The 5-year high-level view can anticipate the major changes in business and technology, while accommodating technical breakthroughs and business shifts when they occur in the near-term detailed plan.

Resistance to Change

As constant as change is in our societies, so too is the resistance to it. Systems planning symbolizes change in many organizations and, as a result, many people avoid it or drag their feet in planning.

In systems planning, much of the lethargy is a result of legacy systems. These are the systems that are currently in place with which everyone has grown comfortable. Many of the people have invested a significant amount of time learning the system. They know how to use it and they know how to get around it. Change in these legacy systems will mean more time invested in learning– time users do not have. Removing these systems can represent a loss in personal competitive advantage and job security. Many of these systems have been significantly customized, and the people remember back to the time when the systems were installed and how difficult that was. Finally, in many organizations the original sponsors, developers, and champions of the legacy systems are still around. Removing *their* systems can be interpreted as finding fault with them or intimating that they are somehow of less value today. Some of this resistance can be overcome by clearly communicating the reason for change and involving those champions in the new effort. Also, in many cases the new system can be designed to take advantage of and leverage the legacy systems rather than going through a wholesale replacement. We embrace this approach that has been successfully used in many hospitals (2) and is the basis for several data repository products.(3)

Academic Orientation

Planning is all too often *not* held in high regard by those who are trying to get a job done. It is perceived as interfering with actual work and, at best, a necessary evil. Those who lead planning assignments can be guilty by association. To paraphrase an old adage: those who can, do; those who can't, plan. It is also often seen as an academic exercise. All too often, it earns this reputation.

Planning often presents, in summary fashion, new ideas and directions. To easily communicate and summarize these ideas and directions, the plan frequently requires charts, graphics, or illustrations. Some planning teams err in trying to communicate too much information in these illustrations (resulting in something that looks like a wiring diagram for the space shuttle). Other planning teams err by oversimplifying the message, creating illustrations that are too abstract or devoid of content. Both results detract from the value of the planning effort. A planning document that is too long or too complicated is ignored; a plan that is intriguing but abstract suffers the same fate.

It is important to keep the team focused on the objective of planning. Planning tends to attract two types of people: those who like to "think out of the box" and stretch the theory; and those that like to test the theory with lots of detail. Both bring value and perspective to the planning effort, but can ruin it if they come to dominate. Careful judgment and balance is the rule of thumb here, with a clear focus on the objective of the plan.

Planning efforts will attract people who like to plan. They will bring enthusiasm and rigor to the effort. This is good. Many of them cannot stop planning. This is bad. There is comfort and safety in planning, and risk and tedium associated with implementation. Many participants will begin to see planning as an end unto itself, receiving inappropriate satisfaction when interim planning products are delivered (e.g., when the rubber hits the sky). This planning merry-go-round or analysis-paralysis can lead to more committees, more task forces, and more planning projects, but rarely to implementation.

We recommend fast track planning. This is an approach that quickly focuses on key functions and early deliverables. A typically *detailed* planning process should take about 20 weeks to complete.

Specific Challenges in Patient Care Information Systems Planning

While each of the previous challenges apply to all systems planning efforts, some unique challenges plague patient care information systems planning.

Medical Culture

Physicians are, at best, demanding consumers. Medicine, as it is currently practiced, is both art and science, and computer systems are expected to support both. Physician independence and unique practice patterns have traditionally frustrated efforts to apply system technology. This has been equally true for the text-oriented documentation needs of nurses.

The technology alternatives and solutions that address the physicians' and nurses' special needs have been discussed in previous chapters. The patient care information system planning process will require significant clinical care providers involvement at a minimum. The more successful efforts have seen clinical care providers in the leadership and design roles. At Brigham and Women's Hospital in Boston physicians have half-time assignments in information planning and design. The Rehabilitation Institute of Chicago and Albany Medical Center both link patient care information system success directly with *early* physician involvement.(4,5) It is also important to involve physicians who have the respect of their colleagues and actually *practice* medicine.(6)

Integrated Care Delivery Systems

As consumers/payers are moving toward managed care and capitation, health care providers are reacting by forming integrated care delivery systems. Horizontal integration links hospitals together while vertical integration incorporates hospitals with individual physicians, clinics, home health agencies, long-term care facilities, and other alternative delivery sites. The implication is that patient care information systems can no longer be designed exclusively for a hospital.(7) They may begin within the facility, but must accommodate all of the constituents of the integrated care delivery system. In the simple case, this means dealing with more legacy systems. In the tougher instances, it means designing around different standards and practices. It may even involve accommodating practice patterns of institutions that are not yet aligned but may be in the future.

The Process

We have discussed what it is, why we do it, and what can get in the way; now we will address *how* to do it. Actually, there is no single correct way to develop a patient care information systems plan. There are several different approaches, each appropriate to certain situations and planning objectives.

Defining the Objective

Most of us understand the value of planning and the need for a "road map." In the real world, however, other needs or objectives may trigger the planning effort. It is important to recognize these objectives, as they can color the process, participants, and products of patient care information systems planning.

Business Change

The need for change may be stirring in several areas within the patient care delivery function. Clinicians or other providers may feel that they are not getting appropriate information support. Department managers may recognize a need to change the care delivery process. Administration may want to address quality or competitive position. In all these instances, there is a motivation to change the status quo. Systems planning can become a political way to initiate change. Planning projects that begin this way must be sensitive to the special agendas of the sponsor. They will also tend to include more organizational and business process redesign aspects in the planning effort.

Self Promotion

In many institutions, information systems may be a "back office" function. Its image is one of technical, pocket protector types, whose job is to run the computer and keep the data flowing. Business decisions are made, strategies are developed, processes are designed, and only then is the information systems department brought in to provide some sort of support. In some organizations this image of information professionals as technodrones is real; in some cases, it is merely perceptual; in some cases, it is a mixture of both. As a result, information systems planning projects are occasionally initiated by the information systems (IS) department to demonstrate the importance of the function, raise the stock of the department, provide exposure for the management team, and earn a seat at the strategy table. This can be an important side benefit of a planning effort, but is a poor driver for the event. When this is the primary motivation, it can lead to grandstanding and self-aggrandizement. Project teams should avoid efforts championed from within the IS function.

Selection

A decision will occasionally be made to purchase a new application system (e.g., a nurse charting system or a point of care system). In the absence of a plan, this decision may appear arbitrary or unjustified. In instances such as this, the sponsor is less interested in a road map than project approval. Before initiating such an effort, the project should be correctly scoped or appropriately labeled as a selection process.

Rationalization

In some organizations no formal information systems plans exist. The strategy exists in the minds of the department managers, the IS director, and the vendor sales reps. The only physical documentation is an occasional memo and the capital budget. At some point an information systems investment decision will be challenged and the decision maker will fall back on initiating a "systems plan." This plan is meant to be a rationalization for a decision already made. Retrofitting a plan to a decision is a useless and frustrating exercise. However, using the need for a decision to launch an unbiased and careful analysis of patient care support needs is a valid objective.

Evaluation

Most organizations will periodically step back to assess where they are. This is common in the information systems arena as well. System evaluations may be initiated to assess the investments made to date. Such an effort may result from unexpected poor system performance. It may result from a perception that there is unused capacity and capabilities. In each case a system audit is usually initiated. Planning projects begun this way have a tendency to be more analytical than strategic and are often detail oriented.

Linkages

Another common driver of systems planning efforts occurs in organizations that have built their own information "tower of Babel." As a result of departmental independence and poor coordination, it has built islands of automation around the institution that do not communicate. The system connections may be either technically too laborious to maintain or organizationally frustrated through departmental rivalries. While the situation would benefit from a cohesive and coordinated plan, the underlying causes of the original situation should be evaluated before starting. Poor direction or coordination in the past can be surmounted through planning. Departmental rivalries, independence and refusal to cooperate, however, will only undermine the subsequent planning effort.

Communications

This is the positive side of self promotion. This motivation recognizes a need for understanding and education for both the system users and system providers. In many instances, planning has been going on informally and this is an effort to formalize the effort and share it with as broad an audience as possible.

Road Map

This is the most common and the best objective for patient care information systems planning. It recognizes that technology must be related to strategy and need. It is based on a need for structure and perspective on this complicated journey. Some elements of this objective are present in nearly all planning assignments. Successful planning engagements will keep it in balance and focus.

Alternative Approaches

Different organizations and different individuals may apply different approaches to patient care information systems planning. No one style is always right. Each approach may be successful depending upon the time involved, detail required, management style of the organization, and objectives of the study. The studies will typically vary along several parameters.

Architecture Versus Selection

After assessing the existing systems and defining the support requirements, some planning studies will move directly to a series of tasks designed to select a packaged software solution. In smaller institutions with limited staff and resources, the easiest path to implementing a patient care information system is to find a single vendor with a comprehensive turnkey solution. In this case, the system and support needs developed at the beginning of the planning study can be turned into vendor evaluation criteria. Moving directly toward the selection task may be the appropriate choice for some smaller institutions.

Most institutions are finding that they are not satisfied with packaged software from a single vendor. Some organizations feel that their objectives can only be met through internal development. In many cases, the optimal solution involves a mixture of internal development and packaged solutions. At a minimum, most organizations find themselves looking at several vendors. In these cases, it is generally valuable to take an architectural approach through a series of views or strategies (e.g., data strategy, functional strategy, and technology strategy). These strategies help the organization understand the relationships between needs and data, data and data, data and applications, applications and hardware, hardware and telecommunications, organization and process, etc. These architectural strategies can be developed at various levels of detail based on the needs of the user. They can provide "30,000 foot" views to see how it all fits together, which can be driven down to the detailed level to understand specific linkages and relationships. As the organization moves into implementation, they become valuable in maintaining perspective and measuring progress. Finally, they become important communication tools that explain design requirements to vendors and process linkages to users.

Retreat Versus Study

Another key parameter is the amount of time and the depth of analysis an organization can commit to patient care information systems planning. Some organizations find themselves with little time for planning. Existing systems may suddenly begin to break down, a rapidly approaching budget or corporate strategy event may demand a systems plan, or a merger/recent acquisition may require a system assessment or rethink. In these instances, plans may be assembled in a matter of 2 to 4 weeks.

Some organizations are comfortable with (or even prefer) short-duration, high-level planning efforts. These are often addressed through planning retreats, a 1 or 2-day off-site session comprised of senior IS management and senior hospital administration. Some high-level communication planning at the one medical center was done over lunch on a napkin.(8)

Most organizations prefer to spend more time understanding the requirements and assessing the alternatives. The additional time also can build more credibility into the results and ownership among the project team and administrative sponsors. Most patient care information systems plans will take approximately 20 weeks to complete. In our experience, system planning projects that run longer than this offer minimal additional value and begin to seriously tax both the interest and momentum of the planning team.

Cookbook Versus Free Form

Another variation in planning approaches is the degree of rigor applied to the methodology. The spectrum runs from the very methodological, with detailed daily tasks and elaborate tracking tools, to the very free-form approach, consisting of only a set of scheduled meetings with loosely defined agendas. For a group with no experience in systems planning, a more methodological approach may be appropriate, as it clearly defines and communicates timeframes, interim products, milestones, and responsibilities. However, there are several risks. The most serious, and the most common, is that the planning team begins to focus on the process and interim products, and loses sight of the objectives. Success, in their minds, is measured by task completion rather than understanding and consensus.

The looser, more free-form approach to planning can be appropriate for a group that has worked together in the past and has enough discipline to get the job done. The risk here is that without some published game plan, the chances are very high for miscommunication and divergent expectations.

There is obviously substantial grey area between these two extremes, and most organizations find themselves selecting an approach somewhere in the middle ground. They will balance the amount of structure according to the management style of the organization and experience of the project team.

Process Versus Directive

This particular planning parameter also closely mirrors the management style of the organization. At one extreme, some planning projects can be very process oriented. Every project team member's opinion carries equal weight. Answers are arrived at through group discovery, and there is a significant focus on building group consensus before moving on to the next task.

Other planning projects can be much more directive in nature. In these projects, a clear leader is obviously directing the effort. Some groups and individual opinions carry more weight than others. Finally, after some discussion, a majority vote or unilateral decision is made, with the result communicated or "sold" to the organization.

Ownership and understanding are paramount to success in planning efforts, and the process approach, done correctly, is typically the better way to engender ownership. It is, however, time consuming. It can be frustrating and in many cases just does not work. For instance, at a Midwestern hospital, an effort at soliciting physician perspective was perceived as railroading a decision that had already been made.(9) As a result, many IS organizations that had developed a myriad of committees to involve the organization are now cutting them back after finding that consensus was never reached. In the meantime, neither decisions nor progress were made.

Obviously, neither approach is effective in the extreme, and most organizations, again, select some middle ground. The pervading successful managerial style at the hospital will naturally shade the approach in the appropriate direction. When in doubt, we recommend working toward a directive approach.

Internal Versus External

This parameter refers to an organization's propensity to use consultants or outside facilitation. Some organizations have the experience and expertise to conduct planning projects with internal staff exclusively. This avoids potential consultant bias, time required to educate the consultant, time required to select a consultant, and obviously the consulting cost. Other organizations place value on the external perspective. The outside facilitator can avoid some internal politics, counter internal bias, and potentially add credibility to the results. If the internal project team lacks experience in system planning projects, the consultant can provide structure, experience, and perspective.

Common Features

While the approach and objectives can vary in the planning of patient care information systems, some components are common to all. These components comprise the plan in its most basic form and can be summarized in terms of six sequential steps. Whether plans are completed in 2 days or 16 weeks, they will generally follow the same path.

Establish Project Scope

At the beginning of each plan there must be an agreement about what the plan will try to accomplish and what aspects are included or excluded from the study. This is important to ensure that the correct approach is used in developing the plan. It is also important for setting expectations among the participants and the eventual consumers or sponsors of the project. Some planners suggest defining success up front.(10)

Assess

The assessment establishes a baseline for change by defining where the organization is today. In a short planning assignment, this may be established subjectively through common knowledge. In more robust plans, it can involve analysis along several dimensions. It may involve assessing where the business is today in terms of current practices, strategies, success measures, etc. It may involve assessing the market, evaluating regional practice patterns, looking at competing organizations, and identifying national trends. It will normally look at the state of current systems support. This can involve a rigorous examination of the technology, the applications, and the support organization.

While assessments deliver many statements of fact, they also provide subjective views. This can include descriptions of the strengths and weaknesses of each area in addition to a comparison with standards and benchmarks.

Define the Need

In its simplest form this involves asking physicians, nurses, and other clinical staff what information support they require. Answers at that superficial level, however, are not particularly useful. It is important to know what they need now and what they will need in the future. Clinical staff are not well equipped to describe system needs.(11) Rather, they are adept at describing how they can and will deliver patient care. A series of sessions between clinicians and information professionals will identify optimal information system support. Process redesign and Total Quality Management tools along with rapid prototyping and "visualization" tools can facilitate this discussion. Once information support needs have been identified, a key challenge is reconciling the conflicting/overlapping needs and the different priorities associated with them. This can best be addressed through individual interviews followed by group process-oriented sessions.

The results of this step can be reported in several different ways. They can be arrayed in long lists that can later be grouped for a selection process. They can be grouped and prioritized based on system status and business strategy. A particularly useful representation involves positioning these information needs on a functional matrix. Using a functional matrix eliminates organizational duplication and helps ensure consistency and integrity in design.

Define Technical Solution

This step involves translating the last two steps ("where we are" and "what we want") into an information technology solution. It starts by identifying a number of technology alternatives. These alternatives are evaluated using criteria derived from the needs assessment and objective-setting tasks. Based upon that evaluation, a single alternative is selected.

This alternative becomes the technical vision for patient care information systems. Again, this vision can be represented in several different ways. It can be reduced to a series of specifications that become the basis for a request for proposal. A better representation can be the series of architectures previously discussed (data, functional, technical, etc.). These architectures provide integrated views of the desired system and can be constructed in varying levels of detail.

Develop Migration Path

With the technical vision finally in place, the migration plan describes how to get there from here. Migration planning can be one of the most difficult steps because it requires individuals to make real tradeoffs. The vision can represent everybody's ideal end-state. With limited resources and funds, however, the organization will have to build to this vision in stages. This means value will be delivered to some staff before it is delivered to others. It means some pet projects may be canceled or redirected. It means coming to grips with the amount of time and money required to achieve this technical vision.

Some organizations cannot step up to the painful realities in migration planning. In these cases the planning process just fizzles away. In other cases the planning team tries to please everybody by setting unrealistic milestones or spending levels. In this case the plan quickly fails in implementation or is recognized as a "pipe dream" and ignored.

While there is no way to entirely eliminate the discomfort in this task, process tools are available to help planning teams prioritize the tasks. An open and logical process will help the team understand the tradeoffs and a directive approach may be required to break deadlocks and maintain a sense of reality.

A good migration plan will have a clearly defined set of tasks with associated timeframes, costs, and responsibilities. Migration planning can be done at several different levels (either high level or detailed) depending upon the organizational need. It can also provide a mix of levels, for example, detailed in the first year and high level for the subsequent 4 years.

Communicate the Plan

This is an often ignored but critical last step. Some institutions treat the plan as an organizational secret, distributing it on a need-to-know basis. Most organizations recognize communication as a key reason for planning. A plan that is done correctly and shared broadly within the organization will set appropriate expectations, allay fears, build interest, and promote discussion.

Case Study: Geisinger®

Organization

Geisinger Health System spans 31 counties in Pennsylvania, primarily in rural areas, and serves more than 2.1 million Pennsylvanians. Established and operated as a multispecialty group practice, Geisinger employs more than 500 physicians at more than 50 different practice sites. Geisinger also operates a 577-bed regional referral center and a 230-bed community hospital. A 99-bed children's hospital is in the final stages of construction. Additionally, Geisinger offers a comprehensive alcohol and chemical detoxification and rehabilitation capability centered around its 77-bed Marworth inpatient treatment center. This integrated health care delivery system provides services through more than 1.2 million annual outpatient visits. Based upon a managed care philosophy, Geisinger's mission is:

> To improve the health of people of the Commonwealth through an integrated system of health services based on a balanced program of patient care, education, and research.

This philosophy has led to the development of Geisinger Health Plan (GHP), a managed care offering with several different product types that cover more than 160,000 members.

Geisinger's clinical information needs are as vast as the geography the organization covers. In any given day, patient flows can entail encounters at multiple sites, covering three different levels of care (i.e., primary, secondary, and tertiary). Manual clinical information flows, even augmented with nominal technology such as facsimile machines, are hard pressed to respond to such patient movement.

As an organization based on a managed care philosophy, Geisinger's patient care information needs must cover the entire health care continuum. Thus, its patient care information system must be able to embrace both inpatient and outpatient activity. Additionally, the patient care information plan must appropriately balance primary care clinical information needs with those of an inpatient setting, including tertiary care considerations such as intensive care units.

Geisinger's information needs for a specific clinical program must be able to support two dimensions. It must accommodate the depth of information requirements for a clinical discipline. It must also support the breadth of information needed to support clinical program integration throughout the organization. Balancing these two dimensions is a difficult challenge.

The major barriers to effective clinical information flow at Geisinger are:

- Geographic spread of the organization.
- Limited internal and external telecommunications infrastructure.
- Lack of definition of balance between primary and specialty care.
- A fragmented existing clinical applications portfolio.

Information Systems Overview

Geisinger's state of clinical information systems at the beginning of the planning effort represented a collection of largely heterogeneous systems that were loosely integrated or interfaced. The inpatient and ambulatory systems did little more than share some basic patient demographic information. The Clinical Laboratory and Pharmacy were the only major ancillaries automated. Radiology had no automation at all. Cardiology had a degree of information systems support that was being extended to other clinical aspects of the Geisinger Heart Center.

An inhouse effort was used to develop Geisinger's Ambulatory Care System (ACS), a system that extracted diagnosis and procedure information from the ambulatory billing system. Clinicians were able to extend the coding for diagnoses and procedures to enhance the level of clinical specificity. Various standard and ad hoc query capabilities were available from ACS.

A comprehensive patient appointment scheduling system had been developed inhouse for use in ambulatory scheduling, but had not been installed at all Geisinger sites. To support this system and the inpatient and ambulatory billing systems, Geisinger established the Patient Extended Database (PED), which serves as a master patient index for the entire organization. Thus, an individual patient has a single Geisinger medical record number, regardless of what site they use to access health care services. PED serves as the central patient database for many different application systems. It served as the model for several other consolidated databases (e.g., providers).

There was no results reporting, other than direct connections to the Clinical Laboratory Information System, nor clinical order entry capabilities. Also, despite having a hospital information system that automated the admission, discharge, and transfer process, this information was not interfaced with other information systems. Thus, redundant data entry of this information occurred.

The technical infrastructure at Geisinger was varied. Multiple hardware and software platforms were being utilized. Although most focus was directed to IBM and DEC, utilizing COBOL and MUMPS, other platforms were present.

The internal telecommunications infrastructure at Geisinger was relatively robust, at least on the central campus. External telecommunications infrastructure were inconsistent due to dealing with multiple providers in a largely rural setting. Although somewhat sophisticated, the overall Geisinger telecommunications infrastructure lacked the maturity to support integrated clinical voice, data, and video transmission.

Decision to Pursue a Patient Care Information System

Geisinger, recognizing the need to improve its methods for communicating clinical information, decided to pursue a patient care information system. The organization understood that it did not have the knowledge or experience to establish a strategy for a patient care information system. Thus, it was decided to engage the services of an information systems consulting firm to assist in the creation of a patient care information system strategy.

The search for a consulting firm was targeted at identifying a firm that had a true understanding of an integrated delivery system such as Geisinger. Although many consulting firms had vast experience in an inpatient setting, few had substantial exposure in a largely primary care environment. Ultimately, a firm was selected that had significant ambulatory care experience in a managed care setting.

Approach

Geisinger's patient care information system strategy was developed as a joint effort by Geisinger clinicians, administrators, information systems staff, and the selected consulting firm. Brainstorming sessions were utilized to establish the various components of the patient care information system strategy.

Multivote processes were performed to determine overall component priorities. The information systems staff was largely responsible for defining the technical and acquisition strategies.

The consulting firm was invaluable in terms of proposing what could be in a patient care information system and facilitating the entire process. It was of particular value in forcing consensus and closure on controversial issues. The firm also played the role of "devil's advocate," frequently providing a reality check when Geisinger staff began to drift from a focused path.

Organizational approval was developed slowly through group participation in the final preparation and wording of the patient care information system strategy. The strategy was then approved by an executive-level information systems steering committee. Following approval, the patient care information system strategy was presented for comment to various clinical forums throughout Geisinger. By the completion of the process, more than 500 Geisinger clinicians and administrators had received copies of the patient care information system strategy, in either detailed or summary form. Many of those individuals attended presentations about the patient care information system strategy as well.

Once broad organization support had been gained for the strategy, acquisition approaches that were consistent with the patient care information system acquisition strategy were discussed. Inhouse development of the overall patient care information system was not considered to be a realistic approach. However, a review of the vendor market offered no comprehensive patient care information system product. Thus, it was decided to select a vendor that offered a reasonable probability of success, and work with them in a collaborative manner to develop a patient care information system.

Strategy Maintenance

The patient care information system strategy has required little maintenance to date. Partially because a significant amount of time was invested during its development, the strategy remains reflective of the overall Geisinger strategy. Resource availability and competing priorities have affected the pace of implementation, yet the relative sequencing of the stages in the implementation strategy remains the same.

Only one topic has created a maintenance issue for the patient care information system strategy, that being an increased interest in telemedicine. The appropriate means to incorporate this technology into the strategy is being explored.

Lessons Learned

Development of the patient care information system strategy at Geisinger was accomplished by making several key "right steps."

- The concept of developing a strategy rather than just "diving in" provided a comfort level for clinicians, management, and staff alike.
- Active participation by multiple constituencies (i.e., physicians, nurses, administrators) provided a broad base for consensus building.
- The use of an appropriate consulting firm offered process facilitation and fresh perspectives on issues.
- The broad distribution and presentation of the patient care information system strategy engaged clinicians in an information systems initiative unlike any they had ever had been engaged in before.

Although Geisinger made several positive moves, in retrospect, it also made some poor ones.

- Although broad input to development of the patient care information system strategy was beneficial, having a broad group actually wordsmith the strategy resulted in highly generic, "middle of the road" document that placated everyone, but failed to definitively deal with some controversial issues.

- There was insufficient participation during the creation of the strategy by primary care physicians (PCPs), particularly noncentral-region based PCPs. This dynamic resulted in a strategy that contained a bias toward inpatient specialty issues.
- The presentation of the conceptual overview and functional strategy sections of the patient care information system strategy were crafted in excessively theoretical terms. Few individuals could readily relate to exactly what the patient care information system was without additional detailed explanation. Such a language and conceptual barrier made it difficult for clinicians to relate easily to the initiative.

Next Steps

Geisinger continues in its pursuit of a patient care information system. It will utilize the patient care information system strategy as its road map on this journey. A collaborative relationship has been established with a patient care information system vendor, and an active pilot project is in progress.

Other specific projects identified within the implementation strategy are being pursued:

- The wide-area network (WAN) has been substantially enhanced.
- The Patient Extended Database (PED) integration has been expanded, including design of real-time integration to maintain its data integrity.
- Real-time admission, discharge, and transfer information is now routinely fed to other information systems.
- The patient appointment scheduling system is being implemented throughout Geisinger.

Successful implementation of a capability to access a clinical repository and utilize intelligent order communications has not been achieved. These initiatives will be the focus of efforts for the immediate future. Additionally, information systems support for Radiology is being pursued. All of these initiatives are also contained within the patient care information system strategy.

Maintenance

A significant amount of effort must go into developing the patient care information systems plan. How do you keep it alive? When the planning is done, how do you keep the results from becoming just another binder that collects dust on the shelf? Too many system planning efforts are consummated with a grand final presentation. The first implementation task is begun amid great fanfare–and then nobody looks at the plan again.

A successful planning effort is one that moves the organization quickly and easily into implementation. It adds consistency and direction to the journey that builds patient care information support. It ensures momentum is maintained and value is received.

There are several strategies that characterize successful planning efforts. Most of these are intuitive, but they will guarantee that the planning effort provides ongoing benefit in directing development.

Keep it Brief

Use of a planning document is inversely related to its size. Successful planning processes internalize the results. When the people who will pay for the system (administration), the people who will use the system (doctors and nurses), and the people who will deliver the system (IS professionals) personally share a common vision, understanding of the tradeoffs, and sequence for implementation–the plan will be successful. The planning document should be a summarized reminder of these agreements that is easy to read and easy to measure/track.

Deliver Results Early

Successful system planning efforts sustain and build momentum. Momentum, interest, and credibility with the clinical users will be linked to demonstrable benefit.(12) In developing a migration plan it is important to recognize this human element and incorporate these benefits early and regularly. This will conflict with a tendency to focus on building infrastructure and solid transaction level systems first. Balancing these conflicting requirements is critical for maintaining interest and progress.

Measure Progress

The lesson from all the quality management activity in hospitals today (TQM, CQI) is that good processes measure progress and become self correcting. Planning is no exception. The migration plan should become a yardstick to measure development.

Revisit the Plan

The plan should be reassessed once or twice a year. More often than that and planning will begin to detract from delivering. Less than annually and the plan may not be consistent with major changes. Revisiting the plan should not be another full planning project to establish a direction though it may realign the direction or refine it by rolling out the next year of detail.

Celebrate Progress

It is important to communicate the plan when it is completed and report progress as it is implemented. Truly successful planning efforts also celebrate progress. Good public relations cannot offset poor results or a faulty system, but they can reinforce good work and sustain interest and momentum through the more tedious portions of implementation. Celebrating progress can involve small rewards, recognition, milestone parties, etc. It helps to communicate enthusiasm as well as advancement.

Maintain Perspective

At the other end of spectrum from ignoring the plan are the organizations that hold to it religiously and refuse to consider changes. For them the plan is not a guide to the journey, it *is* the journey. Success can only be achieved by unwaveringly marching to the migration plan milestones. They lose sight of the objective and begin to serve the plan rather than the care delivery process. Then, when something forces a change in direction (and it always does) the entire plan is considered useless and outdated.

It may seem obvious that this behavior is extreme but for those in the trenches, chartered with delivering on the plan, it can slowly and inconspicuously begin to show up in their behavior. Successful plans carry perspective into the implementation. Managers help the staff keep their eyes on the objective and adapt the plan as needed.

References

1. Gardner, E. Reality hinders efforts to fill info system wish lists. Modern Healthcare, November 1992;40.
2. Curtis EH, Patterson VR. Implementing a clinical information system. Topics in Health Record Manager, August 1991;12:1:10-21.
3. Cavanaugh, F. Information architecture: The repository alternative. Computers in Healthcare, November 1992;16-19.

4. Schreier, J. Physicians who use the system help hospitals gain advantage. Computers in Healthcare, August 1991;30-33.
5. Booker, E. Piecing together a distributed system at Albany Medical Center. Computers in Healthcare, November 1989;20-22.
6. Furry SL, Moeller DJ, Tonnemacher SM. Optimizing physician involvement in information systems. Topics in Health Care Financing, Spring 1990;16(3); 22-27.
7. Nordin, JR. Systems implications of alternate site healthcare. Journal of Systems Management, June 1992;13-17,41.
8. Judge, J. The data debate. Hospitals, April 20, 1993;67:8:28-32.
9. Hard, R. Hospitals Increase Med Staff Use of IS. Hospitals, January 5, 1993;67:1:43-45.
10. Meltzer Wallach, R. A tale of two hospitals. Computer Systems News, May 1990;28-29.
11. Jacobsen TJ, Schleyer RH, Kmiecik Smith R. Better planning needed to strengthen patient-care systems. Computers in Healthcare, October 1992; 20-26.
12. Laughlin, ML. A unique approach persuades physicians. Computers in Healthcare, December 1991;18-20.

6
Implementing the Patient Care Information System Strategy

Jami L. Ritter and John P. Glaser

As with all well-laid plans, the most challenging part of an information system strategy is successfully implementing the plan. But what do we really mean by *implementation* and how do you know that it is *successful*?

When we refer to implementation, we mean far more than merely plugging in the computer and turning on the screen. In our vernacular, implementation is the *process* of introducing an information system throughout the institution *and* ensuring that its full potential (benefits) is achieved. We classify a successful implementation as one that:

- Promotes and supports the institution's ability to execute its business plans and meet its business goals. "Organizations are discovering that successful information systems . . . implementation in the healthcare enterprise requires . . . a firm understanding of the organization's overall strategic plan."(1)
- Improves the overall performance of the institution. The system must be recognized as a "strategic tool and corporate asset [that] can represent an investment in an organization's viability."(1)

For most health care organizations, these business goals and performance improvement objectives are converging to a similar set of priorities. We believe the direction of change in the health care environment is clear. Regardless of the specifics of health care reform, most health care organizations are moving toward:

- Collecting and reporting data on the clinical, functional, and financial outcomes of care processes.

- Implementing mechanisms to effectively and efficiently *manage* care processes.
- Gaining efficiencies in delivering services and in meeting the needs of "customers," such as patients, physicians, payors, etc.
- Developing capabilities to combine and share clinical, financial, and administrative data within the facility and across organizational entities that are part of an integrated care delivery system.

These goals pose fundamental challenges for the design or selection of patient care information systems (Chapter 4) and for the development (Chapter 5) and execution of the information system strategy. In this chapter, we will discuss the approaches to and challenges of implementing a patient care information system strategy in this radically changing environment.

Historical Perspective

Historically, there has been much debate about the best approach to implementation of a new system. One approach has been to introduce the system by department, where a laboratory application, for example, is introduced throughout the institution and then the radiology capability is introduced, and so on. Alternatively, some institutions have taken the approach of implementing the system by nursing unit (or by outpatient clinic) where the entire capability is introduced initially on one unit and then rolled out unit by unit.(2)

In the past, these approaches have been appropriate for institutions that lack an installed base of automation support. For these organizations, the goal was to achieve a basic level of information support. Today, however, health care organizations typically have some level of automation that can be strategically leveraged and built upon.

Furthermore, two dynamics are shaping the need for health care organizations to rethink their approach to information systems planning and implementation (Figure 6-1). First, the pace of change in the health care environment is forcing health care institutions to improve customer service–access, quality, and efficiency–through strategic alliances. To do this, the roles and responsibilities of individuals within the business are broadening. Second, and at the same time, the technology change cycle has developed a momentum and direction for change of its own where organizations are rewriting applications, retooling infrastructures, and revamping the information systems. The result is that the information technology capabilities are not keeping pace with business changes.

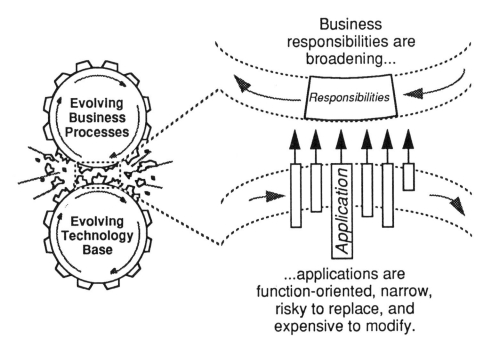

Figure 6-1. Differing Pace of Change Between Business Processes and Technology Base

In this environment, it is no longer viable for health care organizations to approach implementation with a departmental or organizational view. Rather, health care institutions must follow an approach that is *organizationally independent*–one that focuses on how work is performed rather than on how work is organized (Figure 6-2). In this way, organizations can develop business strategies and information systems plans that guide the implementation approach in a way that provides support to critical areas affecting the health care organization's core business–providing patient care.

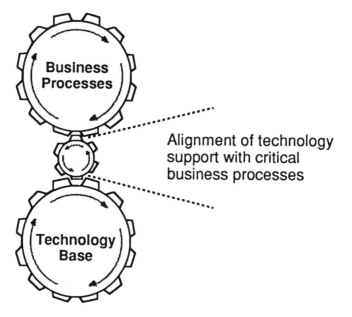

Alignment of technology
support with critical
business processes

Figure 6-2. Technology Alignment to Support Business Processes

Current Thinking

Today, it is generally accepted that the implementation of information systems is a process that must be managed. It is not a one-time effort following a planning process that identifies the need to introduce a prioritized list of applications and their supporting hardware and networks. Rather, the distinction between planning and implementation is becoming much more fluid and iterative. In fact, we believe that both the planning process (Chapter 5) and the implementation process must be managed across three dimensions (Figure 6-3):

- *Strategy.* There must be regular evaluation of the information system's support of business goals and creation of a competitive advantage for the institution. The business strategy should guide the priorities for implementation.
- *Processes.* Critical processes and roles must be evaluated, reengineered, created, or eliminated in an effort to meet strategic business objectives.
- *Infrastructure.* Organizational and technological resources must be flexible, appropriately aligned, and effectively managed to meet changing requirements.

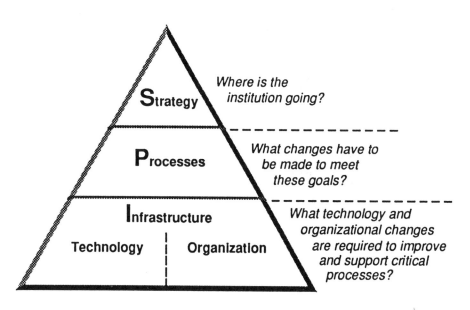

Figure 6-3. Management of Information Systems Planning and Implementation

These three dimensions are essentially enablers or environmental factors that, when aligned, ensure successful implementation. This theme is supported in the literature published within the health care industry as well as by publications from other industries:

- "There's a dramatic need to bridge the gap between the business [strategy], clinical [processes], and technology [infrastructure] sides of the hospital." A series of key action items necessary for achieving this vision are identified:
    – "Develop a strategic vision everyone understands";
    – "Redesign outdated processes";
    – "Manage the culture through change"; and
    – "Invest in a technology infrastructure."(3)

- Another author suggests that strategic information systems planning efforts should strive to:
    – Align information systems investments with business goals;
    – Ensure the efficient and effective management of resources; and
    – Develop effective technology architectures.(4)

- In a banking publication, the author declares that information strategies must be managed across tactical, organizational, and technological dimensions.(5)
- The results of a study published in 1991 identify mechanisms for overcoming barriers to implementing information systems strategies as reported by United Kingdom companies from a variety of industries:
    - Confirm that there is a "formal link" between the information system strategy and the business plan;
    - Ensure that senior management involvement is sustained beyond the planning stage through the implementation stage; and
    - Plan for an evolutionary development of information systems toward more effective information management systems within a technology architecture that relies on common standards.(6)
- Another author estimates that in 1991 U.S. firms were spending approximately $10 billion annually on evaluating environmental trends and formulating business strategies. However, only 10 percent of these plans were implemented as intended. The author postulates that one reason for this failure is that executives do not appreciate the significance of the changes that must be made in "how their organization, people, processes, and systems work in order to achieve the improvements in performance associated with a particular strategy."(7)

We believe that successful patient care information systems result when the implementation is viewed as a series of *business* projects (rather than information systems projects) that are effectively linked to business strategy and to process and organizational changes. Furthermore, these projects are most appropriately led and championed by business people rather than information systems professionals (with the notable exception of technical infrastructure implementations that truly require technical savvy).

Getting Ready

A series of organizational conditions must be in place prior to embarking on an implementation of the patient care information system plan. These prerequisites are essential for getting the organization ready for change and ensuring a successful implementation.

One of the most effective mechanisms is the execution of a change management program. We define change management as a systematic approach that influences behaviors to promote high organizational performance and generate high staff morale over an extended period of time. An effective change management program will ensure implementation of improved processes, minimize operational disruption, prevent staff confusion, and reduce natural resistance to change.

Change management strategies developed by countless experts are often presented as models illustrating sequential step-by-step approaches. Realistically, managing change is a highly integrated, interactive process that supports multiple change initiative activities occurring simultaneously. Managing this complex process requires planning, organizing, facilitating, and communicating activities in a comprehensive fashion that pervades the organization across functional lines, as well as up and down the hierarchy.

The ability to manage change often marks the difference between the success and failure of implementing a change initiative and moving an organization forward. We have identified several critical success factors.

Communicate the vision clearly and frequently. A clear, understandable vision of the future is a key element for managing change. As we discussed earlier, the linkage between the business strategy and information system planning is critical to success. Effectively communicating the vision for this linkage is also paramount. People must grasp the organization's vision and its goals to understand why they should change and the benefits of the change.

Important strategic considerations to communicate include:

- The role of the organization in an integrated delivery system, the characteristics of its partners, and its relationships with these partners (as discussed in Chapter 7).
- Methods and parameters that will be used to monitor, measure, and report on the organization's performance.
- The internal approach to improving and managing care processes, including the composition and governance of committees/teams, resource availability and allocation, project schedules, and expected outcomes.
- The role that information systems will play in supporting the institution's efforts to implement change, achieve strategic objectives, and enable staff to focus on the business rather than on information management tasks.

Begin change management activities early in the strategy development process. Ideally, change management activities should be incorporated into the strategic planning process beginning with the creation of the vision through the implementation of the change.

Foster ownership of the changes and their implementation. People who are most familiar with the work performed in the impacted areas are the logical ones to promote change. Their participation will engender ownership and help gain commitment to smooth implementation.

As we described earlier, radical changes are affecting the health care institution's core business–providing care. These changes have a particularly significant impact on the medical staff. As a result, their leadership is a prerequisite for success. Senior, respected, and politically strong members of the medical staff must fully believe in the need to respond effectively to the changing delivery system and must share the organization's vision for change. This medical leadership must take a proactive role in guiding the institution's response by working closely with the rest of the medical staff, as well as with the nursing and administrative staff to plan effective implementation strategies and to champion use of patient care information systems.

Two particularly relevant experiences described in the literature illustrate this point. In evaluating the success of their system implementation, staff at the Albany Medical Center discovered deficiencies in their change management program. The staff indicated that although they had singled out the change management program as their biggest challenge, they ultimately underestimated the extent of the challenge. One particular deficiency was the lack of appropriate staff in the system selection and implementation process. Interns and residents did not have active input into the process although they became the heaviest users of the system.(8)

In a second example, staff at the University of Virginia Medical Center came to a similar realization. At the conclusion of a traumatic system implementation experience, they concluded that "the implications of the changes should be explained to those most directly affected, and key personnel should be introduced to the anticipated long-term benefits."(9)

Identify barriers to change as soon as possible and plan to manage them. Barriers to change traditionally sort into four categories: strategic, organizational, financial, and cultural. It is important to recognize that although many barriers are obvious and concrete, less tangible barriers known as the "unwritten rules" also exist. These unwritten rules are implicit in the organization's mission statement and corporate guidelines. Staff gain insight through observation of behaviors that are rewarded versus those that are penalized, and staff act accordingly. As an example, an academic medical center might state that the institution's primary mission is to deliver the highest quality patient care, yet the unwritten rule is that career progression and tenure are dependent upon published research.

"For high-performance business transformations to succeed, senior management must ensure that the behavior that naturally follows from the unwritten rules is in line with corporate objectives."(10) There are two alternatives for achieving this imperative: (1) ensure that change initiatives fit within existing rules or (2) modify the rules of the game to support change initiatives. In the example of the unwritten rule for academic medical centers, an effective response would be to ensure that patient care information systems support *both* care and research processes.

Show early results to maintain momentum. Early successes foster enthusiasm and inspire further commitment.

In addition to deploying an effective change management program to prepare the organization, the institution should also have:

Experience with continuous improvement or total quality management (TQM) tools and philosophies. The focus on improving the processes of providing care demands the involvement of cross-functional, multidisciplinary teams. Effective functioning of these teams will be guided by the basic tenets of TQM. It is helpful if the institution has applied these principles in the past and taken the opportunity to tailor them to its particular organizational culture and values.

Solid foundation of information systems investments. To improve performance, participate in new delivery systems, and respond to environmental changes in general, the institution must be able to meet its most basic information needs. Garnering information systems resources to mount a response becomes all the more difficult, if not impossible, if basic information is inaccurate, unavailable, inaccessible, or incomplete.

Assuming these precursors to change are in place, the institution is now ready to implement the patient care information system plan.

Dimensions of the Implementation Process

In today's turbulent health care environment, health care organizations must have shorter planning cycles as well as rapid, responsive implementation approaches that manage the process across three dimensions: strategy, processes, and infrastructure.

Strategy

As we have maintained, a critical success factor for implementing an information system plan is ensuring the link with the institution's strategic business plan. Ideally, the information strategy should be intimately tied with the business strategy. The CIO at Pitt County Memorial Hospital in North Carolina attributed his hospital's success in implementing their information system strategy to "tying the information systems plan to the hospital's overall strategic and fiscal plans . . . [the] information systems plan supports the hospital's strategic plan."(11)

According to R. D. Galliers, "the IS strategy is very much embedded in business strategy: it both feeds off, and feeds into, the business strategy process, which in turn [has] a two-way interrelationship with the company's business environment."(12) This two-way relationship implies the necessity for periodic review and evaluation of the business environment and, in turn, a similar review and evaluation of the business strategy, as well as the information system strategy and implementation plan.

As discussed in Chapter 5, the information system plan typically is developed for a 2-to-5 year time horizon. However, the implementation plan should be created for a shorter time horizon–we generally use a 1-year time frame as the guide. Longer implementations are ineffective in settings where environmental trends are constantly evolving and so too are user needs and technological advances. The implementation plan should be updated annually based on the evaluation of the strategic business goals and the business environment.

The priorities for implementation should be guided by these business objectives as well as by customer needs, and the critical processes and roles that require information support. Let's review each of these priority-setting parameters.

Business objectives. Through an analysis of key customer expectations (e.g., to provide the highest quality care in the most clinically and financially effective manner), critical environmental trends (e.g., the JCAHO information management initiative, the need to measure and report clinical and financial patient outcomes), and the competitive market (e.g., the formation of integrated care delivery systems), a set of business objectives are established for the institution. These objectives are then ranked according to their relative priority.

Key processes and roles. To compete in an institution's chosen market(s) and respond to customer needs, the institution must be able to execute key processes efficiently and effectively and provide adequate information support to critical roles.

A process is essentially a set of activities, with a distinct beginning and end, that results in the delivery of a product or service to customers. Typically, institutions have between 12 and 15 critical processes. Generically, the list of processes for a health care organization could include:

- Planning services
- Marketing services
- Coordinating services
- Assessing patient/planning care
- Delivering care
- Reviewing care
- Scheduling patients and resources
- Documenting care
- Managing costs
- Managing material
- Managing facilities
- Collecting revenue
- Managing information
- Developing staff

The identification of critical processes lays the foundation for defining key roles. We define a role as a set of job characteristics that describes:

- The how–tasks, events, responsibilities, and priorities
- The what–goals, objectives, and targets
- The enablers–skills, accountabilities, incentives, and ownership

More than one individual can play the same role. Chapter 7 describes our view of the roles that will be critical for integrated care delivery systems.

Setting the priorities for providing improved information support will be guided by identifying key roles that have gaps in current information support or opportunities to improve existing information support. There may be new roles that require information support to expand the institution's services, to form strategic alliances, or to meet regulatory requirements.

The final outcome of these analyses is a prioritized list of roles where improved information support can have the greatest impact. By focusing the implementation approach in this manner–on how work is performed–the linkage between business and information management strategies is ensured, and the identification of opportunities to exploit information management to improve overall performance is accomplished. As you may recall, these are the two measures of successful implementation that we identified at the beginning of this chapter.

Processes

Another basic principle of implementing an information management strategy is that the business processes and the information processes that support critical roles should be evaluated and redesigned in concert. In reality, this rarely happens, largely because of timing issues. Most often, information systems are acquired to fit one way of working, but by the time they are implemented, business conditions have changed, priorities have shifted, and user needs have evolved. Furthermore, health care organizations have been notorious for acquiring information support and automating the current way of operating. A case in point is the evolution of nursing documentation systems that support nursing assessments, the Kardex, etc. Many health care organizations have implemented these systems to automate traditional care documentation processes in which *all* care provided is documented. With these systems, the ability to distill and analyze information is hindered by the volume of information and by the lack of standardization. Through evaluation and streamlining of the documentation process, other health care organizations have implemented systems that support charting by exception, where only *deviations from the care plan* are noted. By implementing charting by exception, the institution benefits from significant savings in nursing personnel time spent in documentation activities. Furthermore, documentation by exception also supports the institution's ability to efficiently and effectively gather and analyze information about patient outcomes, costs of care/services provided, etc.

To ensure that information support is appropriate and effective, process redesign and role definition should be an explicit step in the implementation process. Key processes should be examined for opportunities to improve their efficiency and effectiveness. During this examination, opportunities to leverage the support of information systems for critical roles should be identified. Creating an example enduser interface for a critical role can serve to help "visualize" how the new process will flow and how information support can be incorporated to achieve the business objectives (Figure 6-4).

The visualization tool is also extremely effective for use in the change management program, as it crystallizes the planned changes and highlights how they will affect endusers.

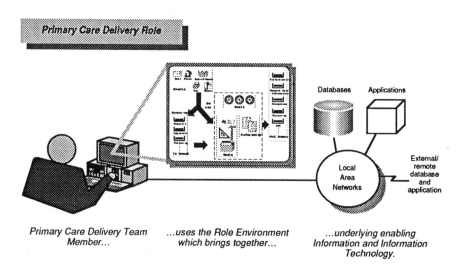

Primary Care Delivery Team
Member...

...uses the Role Environment
which brings together...

...underlying enabling
Information and Information
Technology.

Figure 6-4. Visualizing the Enduser Interface

Infrastructure

The infrastructure has two components: organization and technology. We will review each of these components in turn.

To facilitate the implementation and maintenance of a new information management approach, appropriate organizational characteristics, roles and responsibilities, and processes must be in place. Our philosophy regarding organizational issues reflects our belief that the future information management approach will reflect a distributed computing environment with more information management performed by endusers.

Organizational Characteristics

Although the particular organizational structure should be tailored to meet the individual institution's needs and culture, the literature reveals models that are found in today's hospitals of various sizes.(13)

In small hospitals (fewer than 200 beds), the information systems manager often falls under the direction of the CFO (who essentially functions in the capacity of CIO) (Figure 6-5). Within the department, there are typically three roles: clinical manager, financial manager, and operations manager.

In midsized hospitals (200 to 400 beds), a CIO is in place who reports to the CEO (Figure 6-6). Two managers work under the CIO's direction: an operations manager who takes responsibility for day-to-day operations as well as system development, and a customer services manager who takes responsibility for enduser computing.

The model for large hospitals (more than 400 beds) is similar to that of the midsized hospital except that a third manager is added who takes responsibility for telecommunications activities (Figure 6-7).

As mentioned, these organizational models are characteristic of today's health care institutions. We believe the typical organizational structure of health care organizations of the future (i.e., integrated care delivery systems that are focused on a patient's care and enrollee's wellness) will require a greater focus on enduser, distributed computing. As illustrated in Figure 6-8, these organizations will evolve from simply providing information center management or a "help desk" to providing "customer service" as well to savvy information system users, including physicians, nurses, and allied health professionals who may be geographically dispersed throughout the delivery system. These endusers will take on more responsibility for designing and maintaining their enduser interface (or role environment) as well as their routine and ad hoc reporting capabilities.

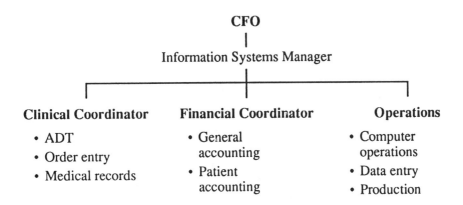

CFO
|
Information Systems Manager

Clinical Coordinator	**Financial Coordinator**	**Operations**
• ADT	• General accounting	• Computer operations
• Order entry	• Patient accounting	• Data entry
• Medical records		• Production

Figure 6-5. Organizational Model for Small Hospitals

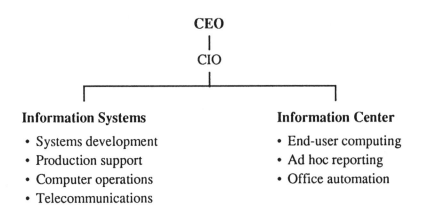

CEO
|
CIO

Information Systems
- Systems development
- Production support
- Computer operations
- Telecommunications

Information Center
- End-user computing
- Ad hoc reporting
- Office automation

Figure 6-6. Organizational Model for Medium Hospitals(13)

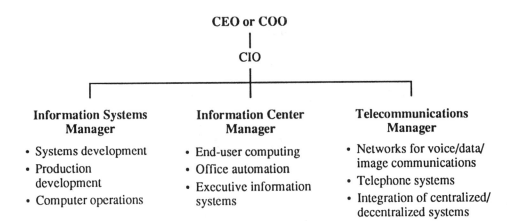

CEO or COO
|
CIO

Information Systems Manager
- Systems development
- Production development
- Computer operations

Information Center Manager
- End-user computing
- Office automation
- Executive information systems

Telecommunications Manager
- Networks for voice/data/ image communications
- Telephone systems
- Integration of centralized/ decentralized systems

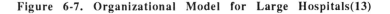

Figure 6-7. Organizational Model for Large Hospitals(13)

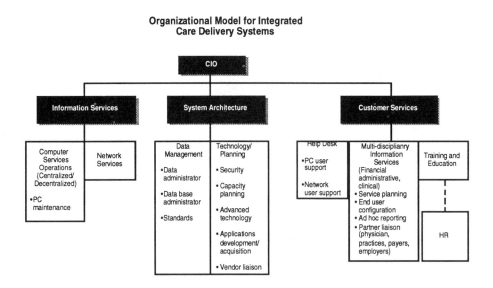

Figure 6-8. Organizational Model for Integrated Care Delivery Systems(13)

In this model, there are three key "middle management" roles under the CIO, any one of which may be filled by the CIO. The Director of Information Services is responsible for day-to-day operations of information as well as network services. The System Architect is responsible for the data, applications, and technology architectures, including maintaining the databases, developing and enforcing data standards, planning capacity, developing and enforcing security measures, and developing/acquiring applications. The Director of Customer Services is responsible for liaison with endusers. The most important responsibility is supporting users in effective information management, which includes working with users to define their needs for information support, designing reports, and reconfiguring and tailoring the enduser interface.

This model reflects the organizational structure of institutions that generally acquire information applications. For those organizations where *development* of applications is a key process, the development team should be located under the auspices of the System Architect.

An organizational structure that is appropriately aligned within the information management culture of the health care organization is critical to a successful implementation. However, the governance plan, which guides processes and activities related to information management, is *pivotal* in determining the ultimate success of implementing the patient care information system strategy.

Roles and Responsibilities

In all models, the role of the CIO is either implicit (as is the case in small hospitals) or explicit. The role of the CIO is to serve as the bridge between senior management and the information systems function. The CIO has overall responsibility for information management services including management of computer operations and networks, systems and architectural planning, and enduser support both within the hospital and across entities in the case of the integrated delivery system model. The CIO is also responsible for ensuring the linkage between the business strategy and the information system plan.

To carry out these responsibilities, the CIO must:

- Understand the driving forces and market circumstances that require the institution to change.
- Participate as a member of the executive team in formulating the institution's responses to these pressures.
- Contribute both business as well as technical knowledge to strategic discussions.
- Encourage the medical staff to provide leadership and to collaborate with nursing and administration staff to carry out the institution's response.
- Manage and monitor the development and performance of information technology initiatives.

To provide the CIO the necessary support structure to carry out these responsibilities, we believe that it is essential to consider the CIO a member of the senior management team. To this end, the CIO should have high-level reporting relationships (either directly to the CEO or to the COO); should be co-located with other senior managers; and should participate on appropriate committees and in routine meetings of the institution's leadership teams. (14)

In addition to the CIO and the core staff within the information systems department, other areas of the health care organization may also develop local information management expertise. These multiskilled information professionals (MSIPs), in addition to their traditional clinical care roles of nursing or medicine, will also develop expertise in planning for and implementing information management initiatives. The MSIPs should remain in their various clinical locations to maintain flexibility to ensure that information management changes support enduser computing needs.

To govern the process of information system planning and implementation, we believe there are three other critical organizational components.

An *Executive or Steering Committee* that takes responsibility for developing institutional strategies, setting information management priorities, and reviewing and approving information management plans.

An *Advisory Committee* composed of representatives of all key processes and roles as well as representatives from other entities that may be part of the integrated care delivery system. This Committee takes responsibility for defining information management needs, developing information management plans, recommending resource requirements, monitoring progress against plans, and establishing enduser/information management partnerships.

Functional teams that take responsibility for improving critical processes within their domain and identifying alternative information management solutions. These teams may already exist (e.g., Infection Control, Nursing Practice) and will take on this expanded role.

Brigham and Women's Hospital, a large, tertiary care, teaching hospital in Boston, Massachusetts, has had noteworthy success in developing and implementing patient care information systems. One of the many reasons for the hospital's success has been the formalization of the relationship between information systems and medical staff. Two committees have been formed that illustrate this commitment to ensuring the appropriate structural alignment.

First, the Center for Applied Medical Information Systems Research (CAMIS) is charged with defining the patient care information system direction, designing and evaluating systems, and assessing the impact of patient care information systems on medical care. CAMIS is composed of four physician-computer scientists (most of whom also practice medicine) and two computer specialists.

Second, the Clinical Initiatives Development Program (CIDP) is responsible for identifying and prioritizing areas where the quality and efficiency of care can be improved. CIDP is staffed by four practicing physicians with strong health services research backgrounds and by representatives from nursing and major ancillary departments.

These committees support the notion that successful implementations require the involvement of senior-level medical staff, particularly given that patient care information systems are being utilized to guide medical care and not merely to report results. Brigham and Women's Hospital firmly believes that strong medical knowledge, preferably provided by physicians, is essential for ensuring the successful design and ultimate implementation and acceptance of patient care information systems.

Although the orientation of Brigham and Women's Hospital is primarily on developing applications, this information management infrastructure is also appropriate for institutions that focus more on acquiring applications. The primary difference is that organizations that buy systems will not require the time intensity nor the number of staff devoted to the process of patient care information system planning and implementation.

Processes

As part of the implementation activity, it will be necessary to define or enhance processes that address project management, prioritization, and monitoring. Although these processes may be in place today and may be traditional activities for the administration and information systems staff, they will most likely be new processes for the medical staff.

As discussed earlier, the involvement of the medical staff is paramount to success. To this end, medical staff must evolve from participants to leaders of implementation projects, from contributors of small blocks of time to contributors of significant time, and from conveyors of ideas to conveyors of medical knowledge

A number of challenges are inherent to this evolution:

- Traditionally, medical staff have worked with information systems staff in an effort to develop systems that support their ability to provide care and that are convenient to their way of providing that care. Today, they must evolve to a role of developing systems that guide and to some extent constrain the way in which they practice medicine and that also monitor their practice of medicine.
- Medical staff must gain appreciation of the strengths *and* limitations of information technology and data.
- Finally, medical staff should become active participants in processes that are comfortable and familiar to information systems professionals but may be foreign to medical staff. Such processes include project management, prioritization, and review.

The CIO can play a significant role in helping the medical staff make these transitions by establishing an appropriate organizational infrastructure that formalizes these new relationships, roles, and responsibilities.

Technology

As discussed in the next chapter (Chapter 7), enduser orientation and client-server technology provide an opportunity to achieve greater flexibility and improved response from information system support. Figure 6-9 illustrates the technology industry's evolution from systems in which the enduser interfaces, applications, and databases are integrated into a single package that is often inflexible and fails to meet the needs of a diverse group of users. Information systems are evolving to separate packages consisting of the enduser interface, the applications, and the databases. These advanced systems will provide the agility, potency, and integration that are prerequisites for successful implementation.

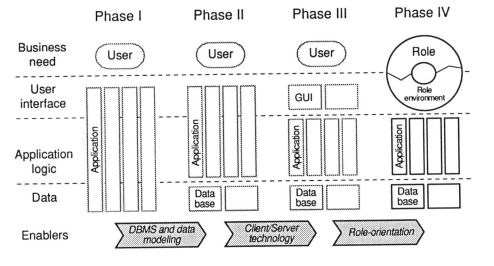

Figure 6-9. Technology Evolution(15)

Progressing from Phase I to Phase IV, institutions gain flexibility in maintaining, updating/modifying, and implementing each of the components.

In Phase I, all components–user interface, application logic, and database–re intimately linked within any single application. As a result, changes made to one component of an application require corresponding changes to the other components.

In Phase II, the database is separated from the linked components of application logic and user interface. This provides an incremental improvement in flexibility in that changes can be made to the database without making corresponding adjustments to the application logic/user interface component.

In Phase III, the user interface is separated from the application logic, which in turn is separated from the database. This is an example of a client-server architecture, which provides a significant improvement in flexibility over Phases I and II. In this phase, changes to any component–user interface, application logic, or database–can be done independently without requisite changes to the other components.

Although Phase IV mirrors Phase III in terms of flexibility and separation of the architectural components, this phase has evolved a step further with regard to the user interface. In this phase, the user interface is designed around the user role (or set of job characteristics) and reflects the user's role environment.

The technology architecture of today's health care organizations is typically representative of Phases I, II, and III. Regardless of which phase the institution finds itself in, however, all organizations should be laying the foundation to implement the Phase IV architecture. Achieving this technical structure should be an evolutionary process that leverages current investments wherever possible and encapsulates current systems that will not be retained long term (only making enhancements when necessary to meet critical business requirements). Furthermore, we believe that, at a minimum, health care organizations should begin to upgrade their networks (particularly their capability to share information across organizational entities), to develop enduser interfaces on workstations for key roles, and to begin building a centralized patient database that integrates administrative, clinical, and financial data at the patient level. The flexibility afforded by this technical structure cannot be overemphasized, particularly in light of today's radically changing health care environment and the need to support increasingly savvy endusers who have unique information needs.

Migrating to Tomorrow's Patient Care Information System Environment

With critical processes and roles identified, an appropriate organizational alignment and governance plan defined, and technology implications understood, the question remains, "how do we get from here to there?" The migration plan is an effective tool for defining the phased evolution from today's information system support to the future patient care information system environment. An effective migration plan should identify all necessary changes, including manual improvements, organizational enhancements, and technical solutions. The changes are phased according to the priorities that the institution has established (relating to business objectives and critical roles in need of improved information support) and according to functional and technical dependencies. For example, a basic requirement for developing a longitudinal patient database that is shared across organizational entities will be the implementation of a registration application with a standardized patient identifier.

Figure 6-10 illustrates a migration plan for an integrated care delivery system. The plan reflects the following changes:

- Applications that should be added, upgraded, replaced, maintained, or encapsulated.
- The patient database that should be developed.
- Network and infrastructure enhancements.
- Enduser interfaces (role environments) that should be defined.
- Operational changes.

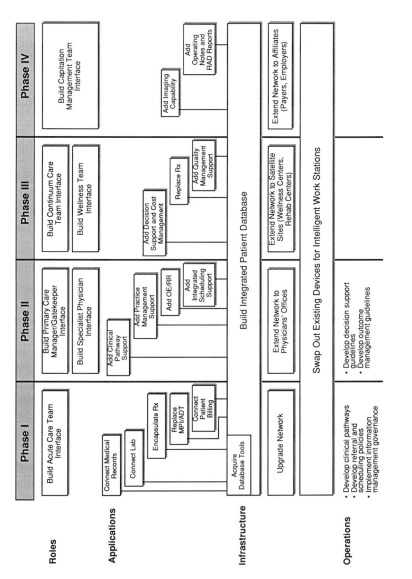
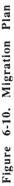

Figure 6-10. Migration Plan

The migration plan should be considered a "living document" that is continually revisited and updated as business objectives change, available technical solutions improve, and user needs evolve.

Conclusion

Implementing the patient care information system strategy differs from other change initiatives in the following ways:

- The necessity for an *effective change management program* cannot be overstated. The practice of medicine is becoming more managed, the measurement of medical practice is focusing on efficiency as well as effectiveness, and the role of senior management in medical practice is increasing. To this end, the evolving role that patient care information systems are playing in the delivery of health care implies a significant change in culture for health care organizations.
- *Deep medical knowledge and the support of senior medical staff* are essential precursors to successful integration of the patient care information system into the routine activities of providing patient care.
- The *planning cycle and implementation sequence must be much shorter* because the health care environment is so turbulent and the specific health care reform picture is unclear.
- The fervor for *technological integration and support for critical processes and roles* is accelerating as health care organizations develop integrated care delivery systems. Departmental systems that support laboratory, radiology, and so forth no longer meet the definition of patient care information systems. Rather, the architectural view must be role oriented to support the health care organization's core business of providing patient care.

Health care organizations can no longer rely on turnkey implementations and assume that their efforts are complete. Implementation, as well as planning, will be a continual effort in which health care institutions must learn to excel to ensure their viability in today's radically changing environment.

References

1. Judge J, London K. The role of the CEO in enterprise-wide information systems planning and implementation. Proceedings of the 1993 Annual HIMSS Conference. American Hospital Association, 1993;237-244.

2. Bria WF, Rydell RL. The Physician-Computer Connection. A Practical Guide to Physician Involvement in Hospital Information Systems. Chicago, IL: American Hospital Association, 1992;39-59.

3. Nelson, I. Leading change: The '90s healthcare challenge. Computers in Healthcare July 1993;14(7):30–33.

4. Earl, MJ. Experiences in strategic information systems planning. MIS Quarterly March 1993;17(1):1-24.

5. Landis, K. Implementing a strategic plan. Banking Software Review Spring 1989;24,26-27.

6. Wilson, T. Overcoming the barriers to the implementation of information system strategies. Journal of Information Technology, March 1991;6(1):39-44.

7. Judson, AS. Invest in a high-yield strategic plan. The Journal of Business Strategy July/August 1991;34-39.

8. Spillane MJ, McLaughlin MB, Ellis KK, et al. Direct physician order entry and integration: potential pitfalls. Proceedings of the 14th Annual SCAMC, IEEE Computer Society Press, 1990;774-778.

9. Massaro, TA. Introducting physician order entry at a major academic medical center: I. Impact on organizational culture and behavior. Academic Medicine January 1993, 68(1):20-25.

10. Scott-Morgan, PB. Barriers to a high-performance business. Reprinted from the American Management Association Magazine Management Review July 1993;37-41.

11. Landis, D. Information systems form large part of strategic plan. Computers in Healthcare February 1991;12(2):23-26.

12. Galliers RD. Strategic information systems planning: myths, reality and guidelines for successful implementation. European Journal of Information Systems 1992;1(1):60.

13. Guide to effective health care information management systems and the role of the Chief Information Officer. Healthcare Information and Management Systems Society Publishers 1994;25-28.

14. Glaser, JP. The role of the chief information officer in creating the clinical information systems infrastructure. Publication pending in the Joint Commission Journal on Quality Improvement.

7
Redefining the Patient Care Information System

Jane B. Metzger and Samarjit Marwaha

The rapidly changing world of health care is ushering in new incentives and business realities that are increasing the urgency of bringing computer-based information tools to bear on patient information management. This chapter describes the driving forces and responses in terms of new models for delivering care and for structuring the health care organization, as shown in Figure 7-1. Collectively, all of these changes increase the need for patient information management and sharpen the definition of the ultimate patient care information system.

They also present new challenges to those responsible for assembling the information and communications infrastructure for an integrated care delivery system. One way of defining the ultimate patient care information system is to examine the key direct care and supporting roles that will be necessary to manage patient health and operate the health care enterprise. This chapter also describes these roles, the information management prerequisites for success in the new health care environment, and ends with a role visualization for a Primary Care Manager/Gatekeeper supported by one view of the ultimate patient care information system.

Health Care Imperatives

Incentives of Capitation

The major driving force for changes in the business of health care in the United States has been the method for reimbursement. Reimbursement in the United States is moving rapidly from the fee-for-service model toward full capitation,

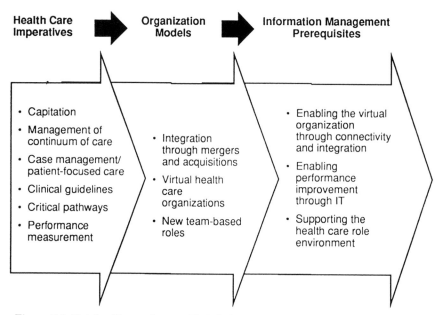

Figure 7-1. Driving Forces that are Redefining the Patient Care Information System

under which comprehensive health care services are provided to large populations of citizens each year for a prenegotiated price, and the health care provider becomes accountable for the health of the covered citizens. This trend toward managed care is advancing rapidly, even without national health care reform initiatives. In some parts of the country, mature (fully capitated) managed care is more common than in others, but the movement everywhere is clearly in this direction.

The four stages of the shift toward managed care shown in Figure 7-2 are progressive, but not mutually exclusive. Currently individual health care organizations are likely to be providing health care services under three (or possibly even four) of the reimbursement modes illustrated. This adds to the complexity of responding to the challenges of the new business, while continuing to meet the reimbursement requirements of the older models.

As health care organizations provide more services under fixed prices or capitation, the business becomes increasingly accountable for delivering uniformly high-quality care at a competitive cost. Accomplishing this requires:

- Managing patient wellness and, during episodes of illness, providing the services that are appropriate.
- Managing the cost and quality performance of all care processes and outcomes.
- Eliminating the barriers to providing care efficiently and in the most cost-effective setting.

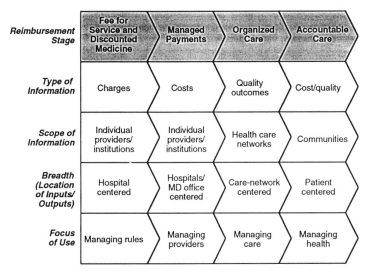

Reimbursement Stage	Fee for Service and Discounted Medicine	Managed Payments	Organized Care	Accountable Care
Type of Information	Charges	Costs	Quality outcomes	Cost/quality
Scope of Information	Individual providers/ institutions	Individual providers/ institutions	Health care networks	Communities
Breadth (Location of Inputs/ Outputs)	Hospital centered	Hospitals/ MD office centered	Care-network centered	Patient centered
Focus of Use	Managing rules	Managing providers	Managing care	Managing health

Figure 7-2. The Shift from Fee-for-Service Reimbursement to Managed Care and Related Needs for Information Support

Each of these prerequisites has a profound effect on the processes and management of health care delivery, as well as on the structure of the health care organization best suited to deliver care according to the new model.

Patient Management

Success within the new model of health care requires managing patient health to maximize health status while providing care effectively and efficiently. Capitation puts the provider (the integrated health care delivery system) financially at risk for each patient's utilization of resources. This results in new incentives to focus on preventive medicine and manage wellness, as opposed merely to respond to incidents of illness. New models for delivering care in a way that meets these goals are patient-centered, driven by an understanding of best clinical practices. Case management/patient-focused care, guidelines, and clinical pathways, discussed in the following sections, are inter-related tools that are being implemented to maximize patient management.

Case Management/Patient-Focused Care

Case management designates one member of the care team with the responsibility for managing all of the services and interactions among team members required for a patient's care. The goal is to coordinate and monitor services across functions and settings so that all necessary interventions and assessments occur when they are needed by the patient rather than in a fragmented process driven by the schedules of departments and the availability of individual team members. In addition to monitoring all services to stay abreast of what is going on at all times, the case manager assesses patient status and progress so that unmet needs are identified or the plan of care is modified by the physician and other members of the care team. In this way case management is intended to ensure that the "right things" are always being done at the "right time."

Case management can be applied to a period of hospitalization or more broadly to managing the continuum of health care services from home to hospital, from hospital to home, or to any other setting where a patient receives direct care. In the broader definition, a case manager implements and monitors referrals across settings, coordinates among physicians and nurses/teams in each site, and may also coordinate with and provide information to payers, employers, etc. Case managers need up-to-date information about patient status and ordered services at all times, in addition to the ability to communicate with responsible physicians and other care providers in each department and setting in which the patient receives care.

Changes to promote a patient focus in care processes can also involve rethinking how the processes that deliver diagnostic services and treatments to patients are organized and where they are located. One approach to bringing services to patients more efficiently involves physically relocating functions such as admissions and some aspects of laboratory, radiology, and pharmacy services out of the traditional departments to patient care areas. This is often accompanied by cross-training of nursing and other staff to perform a broader range of patient care tasks. The point of these changes is to bring the services to the patient, rather than vice versa. Our recent survey of hospitals that had reorganized to implement patient-focused care revealed that most found existing patient care information systems could not be configured to meet the needs of patient-focused care.(1)

Clinical Guidelines

The rationale behind developing clinical guidelines is that unnecessary variation in clinical practice affects both the cost and quality of care. Guidelines are an attempt to define best practices and improve patient management decisions by making physicians more aware of optimal strategies for diagnosis and patient management. If they succeed, guidelines should lead to a more uniform quality of care and more consistently effective application of health care resources.

Increasing interest in clinical guidelines has lead to a number of public and private efforts to develop guidelines. In 1989, Congress created the Agency for Health Care Policy and Research (AHCPR) and charged it with arranging for and overseeing the development of "clinically relevant guidelines" for use in guiding and monitoring care to Medicare and Medicaid patients.(2)

A large number of physician and nursing professional organizations have also developed guidelines, and the American Medical Association directory published in 1993 contained more than 1,400 of these.(3) Health maintenance organizations have also been developing guidelines to address an increasing number of patient management topics identified as opportunities for improvement. One published report that has emerged from this effort suggests the following criteria for choosing topics:

> common clinical conditions; unexplained variation in clinical practice; variation in internal or external referral patterns; general clinical uncertainty or controversy; uncertain indications for risky or costly intervention; internal resource access or supply constraints; apparent risk management problems; introduction of a new diagnostic test, therapeutic procedure, or medication; and quality of care problems perceived by patients, clinicians or managers.(4)

More than 30 percent of hospital executives surveyed in 1993 indicated that patient management initiatives in their hospitals included development of practice guidelines.(5)

Clinical Pathways

Critical path methodologies originated in the construction and engineering fields where they have been used for many years to manage large, complex projects. The underlying principle is to maximize performance (quality and efficiency of production), while minimizing delays and resource utilization through identifying an optimal sequence and timing of activities for a given process and actively managing each step of production against these expectations.

As applied to health care, clinical pathways (also called critical pathways or care pathways) represent the typical or expected progression of interventions and improvements in patient status for a particular diagnosis. They define an optimal sequence of all health care interventions, integrating those of physicians, nurses, and other providers into one map or outline that charts the anticipated patient course over an expected time line of discrete time periods. For each time period, the pathway reflects the problems to be resolved, the health care interventions, and the intermediate goals and outcomes.

Clinical pathways, practice guidelines, and case management are often implemented hand-in-hand. The care pathways for specific diagnoses are generally laid out by interdisciplinary teams, based on a consensus concerning best practices from clinical guidelines and experience. Implementation usually involves case managers coordinating interdisciplinary care teams who manage each patient according to the map of expected interventions and progress, as laid out in the pathway and adjusted as necessary to fit each patient. When patient variances (deviations from the anticipated course of care) are documented and analyzed, clinical pathways can be continually assessed and revised to improve outcomes or efficiency.

Clinical pathways typically are developed first for high-cost, high-risk, or high-volume diagnoses and procedures in order to reap significant savings in resources and improvements in patient outcome, but they eventually will be applied to patient care much more broadly. Initially, the type of health care episodes covered in clinical paths are inpatient admissions. In one survey conducted in late 1993, 44 percent of hospital executives reported that formal initiatives were underway to develop and implement clinical pathways for inpatients.(5) Eventually these tools are expected to be used to guide management of episodes of patient illness across all settings of care (prehospital, follow-up institutional and outpatient care, and home care).

Measuring Performance Through External and Internal Report Cards

Holding providers of care accountable for both cost and quality means that performance is measured as the value the investment purchases. Informed decisions about where to obtain the best value require these new measures of performance to make comparisons among providers. Payers, employers, and the public increasingly expect to be able to judge performance through comparative data.(6) Performance monitoring is also shifting from the traditional focus on inpatient services to address ambulatory care and expanding to include measures of wellness and patient satisfaction with services. The Health Care Financing Administration has initiated the DEMPAQ Project to develop performance measures for clinical events and actions in physician office management of Medicare patients.(7)

Employers and other payers are requesting performance data from managed care providers.(8) The *H*ealth Plan *E*mployer *D*ata and *I*nformation *S*et (HEDIS) 2.0 developed by a national coalition of health plans will be adopted widely within the managed care industry.(9) Another initiative sponsored by 23 vertically integrated health care systems is testing 12 measures that are to serve as the starting point for an ongoing performance measurement system for integrated health systems.(10)

Some states have mandated periodic reporting of performance data (the so-called health care report card), and most proposals for national health care reform include similar mandates. Accrediting bodies such as the National Council for Quality Assurance (NCQA) and the Joint Commission on Accreditation of Healthcare Organizations (JCAHO) are also seeking information to determine level of performance. NCQA is using the HEDIS indicators in its new accreditation process for managed care organizations. The JCAHO's Indicator Measurement System (IMSystem) will use continuous collection and periodic feedback of performance measures defined as clinical indicators to complement the standards-based accreditation process.(11)

Integrated delivery systems will be motivated to continually monitor their results on external report cards because these will be the basis for competition in the marketplace. Under full capitation, they are also at financial risk to maintain wellness and manage illness effectively. Therefore, to manage the business, they will need information on how key processes are operating and the results being achieved by the investment of health care resources.

In order to improve performance, integrated care delivery systems require the ability to reexamine care practices continually to pinpoint unnecessary variation and identify potential improvements in effectiveness or resource utilization. In order to target areas for improvement, they will need performance data that identify differences in the provision of care among their sites and providers. They also must be able to benchmark performance against local competitors (for cost and value) and nationally recognized leaders with best practices (for quality). (The JCAHO IMSystem is intended to support both internal improvement efforts and benchmarking against a national reference database.) Thus, the successful health care enterprise will continually reassess how it provides care using many different versions of "an internal report card."

Emerging Organization Models

Integrated Care Delivery Systems

The trend toward managed care and reimbursement via capitation is creating new relationships among health care entities. The imperative to provide seamless, high-quality care will require innovative approaches to organizing the delivery of health care. Today, no one organization can ensure wellness and provide care across the entire continuum of services. In place of the traditional structure of hospitals and independent physician practices, new entities are emerging that can offer integrated services encompassing both physician and hospital care and engage in full-service contracts to provide comprehensive services to meet the health care needs of a defined population of citizens.

Integrated care delivery systems are a natural consequence of the new health care environment because they provide the organizational structure that is best suited to ensure good outcomes at the least cost. Because integrated systems include the broad range of health care settings, care can be provided in the setting(s) that minimize the cost per episode. Because they incorporate the primary care setting, integrated care delivery systems are in a position to manage patient health through preventive care and manage care delivery through episodes of patient illness. They are also able to manage care across traditional organizational barriers that have made it difficult to coordinate and ensure continuity of patient care.

At the simplest level, the new integrated care entities are Physician-Hospital Organizations (PHOs), jointly owned organizations of physicians/physician groups and hospital(s)/hospital systems. Another likely scenario is that these organizations will share risk and information to become a mutually dependent virtual organization. Such a virtual organization will have lower administrative overhead and greater flexibility, while enabling individual institutions to maintain excellence in their areas of specialty. Other models, such as joint ventures and full integration, have more formal integrating structures for achieving the same objectives. In many cases the integrated delivery system incorporates other entities such as long-term and rehabilitation care facilities and home care services.

This joining of health care entities into integrated care delivery enterprises is occurring rapidly. A survey of health care executives in late 1993 indicated that 57 percent of hospitals, 77 percent of multihospital systems, and 45 percent of physician group practices have already created integrated delivery networks according to one of these models, or are expected to do so by the end of 1994.(12)

Emerging Roles

As providers share in the risk of capitation, they will assume broader responsibilities and demand greater access to information across the continuum of care. For example, a primary care physician at risk will feel much more accountable for (as well as have a vested interest in) not only the care he or she provides but also what happens after a referral, wellness within the home or work, and the effectiveness of protocols, drugs, etc.

Inevitably, broad roles that are highly dependent upon information will evolve within the virtual health care organization, as shown in Figure 7-3. Staff playing all of these roles will feel the need to provide the best patient-focused care, not just to be the best in their disciplines. Although the focus of most roles will be delivering care, the additional roles shown in Figure 7-3 that enable efficient delivery of care and managing the health care enterprise will also be critical.

Roles may manifest themselves differently in health care organizations. For example, the physician who serves as the Primary Care Manager/Gatekeeper may also be a member of the Wellness Team. Likewise multiple management roles might be combined in initial, smaller integrated care delivery systems, while in larger enterprises each role may be performed by a cross-functional, cross-organizational team. Ultimately, however, each of these roles must be filled for the health care enterprise to prosper. Collectively, they provide a framework for information planning and defining the ultimate patient care information system.

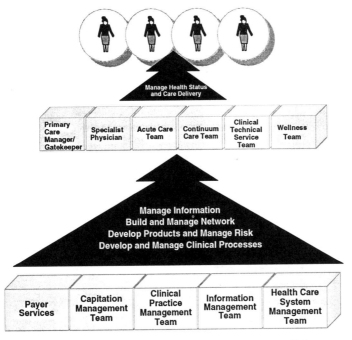

Figure 7-3. Direct Care and Supporting Roles that Provide the Infrastructure for Managing Health Status and Care Delivery

Direct Care Roles

Care professionals will assume one or more of six distinct roles (shown in the upper half of Figure 7-3) to manage the health of the population under the care of the integrated care delivery system. The share of the patient care planning, implementation, and monitoring responsibilities of each role will determine the nature of their needs for information access and management.

The *Primary Care Manager/Gatekeeper* will act as each patient's entry point into the health care system, providing basic primary care services and managing all referrals to specialists, diagnostic services, and acute care settings. For this role, physicians will need:

- Up-to-date patient information.
- Assistance in managing patient problems according to local clinical guidelines and best practices through care pathways and decision support available at the point of care.
- The ability to coordinate scheduling of other services in the most efficient settings.

To manage each patient between encounters, physicians playing this role will also need assistance with following up on all outstanding tasks and services, and effective communication with referral providers and institutions, the Continuum Care Team, and the Wellness Team. Periodically, each Primary Care Manager/ Gatekeeper will receive feedback on performance measured against standards as input to continual improvement in care practices.

Upon the referral of a Primary Care Manager/Gatekeeper, *the Specialist Physician* will manage a single episode of care or, for a chronic problem, manage a patient on a recurring basis. The specialist will be responsible for managing the episode of illness according to locally determined best practices for the specialty/subspecialty of practice and against the resource map and anticipated time-phased patient recovery, as defined in a care pathway for the diagnosis(es). To play this role successfully, the Specialist Physician will need:

- Effective communication with the referring provider.
- Current information on patient status.
- Assistance in matching the patient with the appropriate protocol or clinical pathway to develop a plan of care.
- Coordinated scheduling of diagnostic and treatment services.
- Assistance with following up on all outstanding tasks and services until the underlying illness or problem is resolved and the episode of referral care ends.

At this point, the Specialist Physician will need assistance in transferring ongoing patient management back to the Primary Care Manager/Gatekeeper and the Wellness Team in a seamless process.

When patients are hospitalized or require day surgery or treatment such as chemotherapy or dialysis, *the Acute Care Team* will manage the discrete episode of care in accordance with established clinical pathways. To perform this role effectively, the Acute Care Team will need to obtain the clinical rationale for the admission from the Primary Care Manager/Gatekeeper or Specialist Physician, up-to-date information on patient health status, and the ability to match each patient with appropriate clinical pathways established for the diagnosis or procedure and to tailor (possibly merge) standard pathways into patient-specific care plans to fit particular needs.

A designated member of the care team will assume a coordination role–that of the patient case manager. The case manager will need assistance in ensuring that appropriate resources are brought to bear, coordinating and monitoring all care activities, and assessing patient status and progress measured against the expectations established in the care pathway. When the patient's course deviates, the case manager will need the ability to modify the care pathway to reflect any modifications (or a new pathway) directed by the care team. When the episode is completed, the Acute Care Team will need assistance in accomplishing a smooth transition of patient management to the *Continuum Care Team*, the Specialist Physician (if needed for follow-up), or the Primary Care Manager/Gatekeeper.

When patients need to be transferred to another setting for continuing care (home care, nursing home, rehab hospital), the *Continuum Care Team* will assume responsibility for ensuring continuity in care and resource management. Doing this successfully will require the ability to manage each patient according to an appropriate clinical pathway, track patient status and progress across settings, and coordinate the appropriate health care resources in each. When the patient no longer requires ongoing services, the Continuum Care Team will transfer patient management back to the Primary Care Manager/Gatekeeper and Wellness Team.

The *Wellness Team* will take responsibility for ensuring that patients are informed and educated about their responsibilities for maintaining wellness and that all relevant health risk factors are identified and addressed. Individuals playing this role will need assistance in identifying all new members of the covered population. Each member needs a wellness assessment, with follow-up of any needed preventive measures (health screening, immunizations, etc.) as defined in wellness protocols and to be scheduled as necessary with a Primary Care Manager/Gatekeeper to address active problems. The Wellness Team will need assistance in identifying and contacting patients to remind them to obtain preventive services and to provide health promotion programs for education and outreach on an ongoing basis. The Wellness Team is likely to work at employer sites, schools, and community settings outside of the health care organization and will need access to patient information, as well as the ability to document patient problems and wellness interventions from any location.

Another role, the *Clinical/Technical Service Team*, will be responsible for providing the services such as laboratory testing, radiology examinations, and physical therapy that are mapped out in each patient's care pathway. These roles are likely to be shared by personnel, some of them located in patient care areas and some of them in separate departments with specialized equipment and facilities. A major goal in providing these clinical/technical services will be coordinated delivery that is "just in time" based on the management plan for each patient. To accomplish this, the Clinical/Technical Service Team will need assistance in accomplishing patient-centered coordination and scheduling, in managing their work flow so that all assigned interventions are completed in a timely fashion, and an effective means of obtaining information from and providing results to any physicians involved in the patient's care and other members of the Acute Care Team.

Business Management Roles

Managing the new health care business will also be accomplished by managers and supervisors in each integrated care delivery system playing one or a combination of the roles in the bottom half of Figure 7-3. Success will require that each role player has flexible access to complete, accurate, up-to-date information about both the clinical and financial aspects of the business, although the specific mix of information and the views of the business will vary according to the management purview of the role.

The *Health Care System Management Team* will be responsible for overseeing the integrated care delivery system, including strategic direction, operations, and financial and resource management. To do this they must be able to take the pulse of the business at any point in time, using a broad range of internal and external standards and benchmarks to monitor performance and identify areas for improvement. This will require access to detailed clinical, resource, financial, and cost information concerning services delivered anywhere in the integrated care delivery system for subgroups of patients, payers, health plans, etc. They must also be able to benchmark clinical and financial performance against that of competitors in the marketplace and thought-leader institutions with best practices in managing successful integrated care delivery systems.

The *Clinical Practice Management Team* will be responsible for implementing and overseeing best practices in patient management. To accomplish this, team members will need to keep abreast of research on clinical practices and guidelines/protocols development by professional associations, governmental bodies, and thought-leader health care organizations. Working with internal, multi-disciplinary committees, they will transfer this knowledge and continually refine internal protocols and clinical pathways to incorporate best practices. They will need assistance in integrating protocols and care pathways into routine patient management at the point of service in all care settings within the health care delivery system and the ability to analyze deviations from care pathways for opportunities to achieve better outcomes through refinement of care practices. To encourage effective clinical practice, they must be able to provide feedback on the practices of different health care sites, departments, and individual providers.

The *Capitation Management Team* will establish and manage the internal and external care delivery network and negotiate and manage contracts with payers for providing comprehensive services to defined patient populations. To do this effectively, individuals playing this role must have detailed information on covered populations and on resource utilization as the basis for negotiating terms of contracts and for monitoring the performance of the network in providing services under each contract.

Payer Services will manage reimbursement from and reporting to external payers. They will need the ability to analyze and provide information on the volumes and types of services provided to each payer, the care practices/pathways employed, and overall performance measured as utilization and clinical outcomes including wellness of the covered population. They will obtain, analyze, and monitor patient satisfaction with services as one important measure of quality.

The information infrastructure that enables the health care delivery system to function as a "virtual organization" will be the responsibility of the *Information Management Team*. This will require putting in place and maintaining systems and communication technology that incorporate patient care pathways at the point of service, capture the necessary documentation as a byproduct of the care process, and provide comprehensive data access and flexible analysis tools to supply the information needed to manage the business of the integrated care delivery system so that it meets its strategic objectives.

Information Management Prerequisites

The ability to assemble and maintain an information and communications infrastructure and to manage information will be essential for the very existence of an integrated care delivery system. There are several major challenges in accomplishing this:

- Enabling all of the disparate departments and entities that make up the integrated care delivery system to function effectively as a "virtual organization" through connectivity and integration.
- Enabling continuous performance improvement through Information Technology.
- Supporting the health care role environment.

These challenges are discussed further in the following sections.

Creating the Virtual Organization Through Connectivity and Integration

Health information networks are needed to tie the disparate entities such as hospitals, physician practices, and home care agencies into a common information infrastructure. Hospital-physician electronic networks increasingly provide the patient information linkages that permit PHOs to function effectively.(13) For larger integrated care delivery systems, wider health information networks are also being put in place to link all of the entities in the enterprise with each other and with other parties such as pharmacies, banks, payers, and employers.

One survey of hospitals completed in August 1993 indicated that 57 percent of them already had electronic links established with of their own medical staff and most had plans to expand this type of electronic network during 1994. Twenty percent had expanded participation beyond the medical staff to other referring physicians in the community, affiliated hospitals, and clinical laboratories.(14)

The need to provide seamless access to care and optimize patient management across all settings means that integrated care delivery systems must have an information infrastructure that captures and provides all needed information anywhere a patient may be treated. Seamless information management requires integrating patient information in addition to enterprise-wide access anywhere the patient is being managed. At the core of the future system a comprehensive, patient-centered database of information is needed that describes the health risk factors, health status, and health encounter history of each citizen in the covered population.

To respond to requirements for external report cards and to support practice analysis for internal management, delivery systems must be able to aggregate and iteratively analyze detailed information concerning all patients and encounters in any setting. Through interfaces of existing systems that capture patient information and integrating technology such as clinical data repositories, integrated delivery systems are developing comprehensive, shared patient databases that can support these needs.

Enabling Continuous Performance Improvement Through IT

Physicians, nurses, and others performing the direct care roles of the emerging health care system will never be able to successfully implement new models for patient management without information assistance. The information task is too great.

For one, there are already large numbers of guidelines, and both new guidelines and revisions/refinements to guidelines will continue to emerge. Within each integrated care delivery system, the Clinical Practice Management Team will determine which clinical guidelines to adopt and under what clinical circumstances recommended guidelines and clinical pathways are appropriate. Over time the set of accepted guidelines within the care delivery system and the criteria for matching with clinical situations will also evolve.

To have any effect on medical decision making, clinical guidelines must be incorporated into clinical practice. Several different techniques have been tried without providing clear evidence of the best approaches, although local consensus among medical leaders and providing feedback to caregivers appear to increase adoption in actual patient management.(15) We feel that access to information also plays a critical role.(16) It is unrealistic to expect staff playing direct care roles throughout the integrated care delivery system to keep up with, remember, and consistently apply the moving target of accepted good practices without complete patient information and patient-specific recommendations at the point of service. As discussed previously in Chapter 1, there is accumulating evidence that this type of information support increases the probability that guidelines will be followed.

The implementation of clinical pathways is also facilitated by information support. Hospitals typically begin their clinical pathway efforts in a modest way, developing pathways for one or two high-volume surgical procedures. Pathways are implemented in a limited number of inpatient units, using paper forms. This approach is useful for gaining acceptance of the concept, but it breaks down when extended to many diagnoses (the task of creating and maintaining the protocols becomes too time consuming) and when patients require several different pathways to be integrated to create a plan of care. Tracking and analyzing patient variances is also difficult with data from paper forms. For these reasons, clinical pathways cannot be implemented widely without information system support.

Another critical element in continuous practice improvement is the need for internal and external report cards. If the Clinical Practice Management Team is continually to reevaluate clinical practice in order to identify opportunities to achieve better outcomes and more effective application of health care resources, they need access to detailed information about the care delivered and tools for identifying the leverage points for improvements. They also must be able to review practice concurrently (in time to intervene) rather than long after the care episode ended.

Collecting data for multiple outcome measures at intervals during the course of patient care is not feasible with traditional tools that extract data from patient charts and key it into computers for analysis. As discussed in Chapter 1, the cost is prohibitive and the information incomplete and error prone.

A 1993 survey of 51 Chief Information Officers (CIOs) from leading medical centers and integrated care delivery systems revealed that though 78 percent were measuring cost outcomes for hospital stays, only 45 percent were measuring cost outcomes across the spectrum of care. Eighty percent were measuring some health-related events (probably mortality and length of stay), but only 16 percent were using HEDIS indicators, and only 12 percent were measuring functional health status. Sixty-five percent were already measuring patient satisfaction, however.(17)

One of the lessons learned by these CIOs was that once the capability to analyze outcomes was introduced, they could not meet the demand for outcomes data. Their computer systems were not capable of handling the processing demands, and they did not have sufficient staff available to structure and run the requested analyses.(17)

Health Care Role Environment

The role environment approach offers many advantages in providing IT support in a rapidly changing business such as health care. Chapter 6 reviewed using role-based views of the business to bring the necessary future focus to redesigning business processes in conjunction with change management and evolving the system architecture to provide flexible, role-oriented support to end users. The "role environment" approach can support the changing health care business on a sustainable basis.

Role environments provide a new way to integrate business and technology by providing a harmonizing agent that synchronizes the technology and the work of the business.(18) The client-server technology discussed in Chapter 6 allows the business to decouple the information screens from the underlying applications. Role orientation allows screens to be coupled with the roles they support. The role environment is a workstation-based user interface that is custom-designed to support a specific business role. It serves as a window into all underlying applications and workflow/communication services.

The successful role environment is multifaceted:

- Provides users with easy access to all of the applications they need, regardless of where the application resides (locally, across a Local Area Network, or remotely across a Wide Area Network). A control-panellike user interface acts as each user's private command center, providing all support including spreadsheets, word processors, and electronic mail.
- Helps users achieve their work goals, not just access data. The role environment is a trusted adviser, not just a "yellow pages."
- Provides for distribution, communication, and monitoring of work. Given the trend toward multifunctional teams in all types of business, a role environment helps to allocate work, route work, monitor the status of work, and escalate the attention it gets when necessary.
- Serves as a conduit for common services. The role environment brings appropriate functionality to the role, rather than yet another application, using common application and system services throughout.

The role environment approach is ideally suited to health care.

- *Supports evolving roles.* As integrated care delivery systems evolve and mature, we will see roles take on new responsibilities or responsibilities will be reallocated. For example, the Primary Care Manager/Gatekeeper is likely to take on responsibilities for implementing wellness protocols during office practice. Care teams will increasingly adopt new models for patient management and extend these approaches more broadly across patient populations and settings. As this occurs, role environments can easily be refined and expanded to keep pace with rapid changes in the allocation and definition of job content and approach.
- *Enables virtual organizations.* As more components join integrated care delivery networks, the role environment approach makes it possible to plug appropriate applications such as scheduling and clinical decision support into workstations for users in the expanded enterprise. This facilitates quick linkage and integration into the electronic network and information backbone of the care delivery system.
- *Puts information to work.* To perform job roles effectively, people in health care, as in other businesses, do not just want access to information; they want information that is relevant to the work they are doing. Care teams managing patients according to clinical pathways need a patient-focused gathering and coalescing of information for each time span in the pathway and the ability to easily track progress toward and transition to the next time period. Communicating via electronic mail and fax is a common aspect of many job

roles. The role environment approach permits combining applications tailored to the job and common functions into a customized interface that puts information to work.

Role Visualization of the Primary Care Manager/ Gatekeeper

The ultimate patient care information system needs to support all of the roles in the emerging health care environment, by providing a customized workstation interface to support each of the direct care and supporting roles as depicted in Figure 7-4.

To conclude this discussion of the ultimate patient care information system, we describe a scenario developed for the Primary Care Manager/Gatekeeper, one of the critical roles direct care providers will play in the new health care environment. Role Visualization is a technique we have been employing to make the discussion of a work role come alive and to illustrate the potential contributions of information support. Screen shots from a role visualization of the Primary Care Manager/Gatekeeper are used to illustrate the information management input from the ultimate patient care information system as the physician playing this role does his/her routine work.

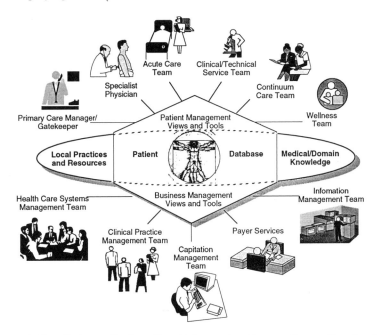

Figure 7-4. The Ultimate Patient Care Information System Supporting the Role Environment of Health Care

Walk Around the Desktop

Dr. Stanlea Livingston's Care Station always displays her daily schedule of patient appointments, committee meetings, and personal obligations. (Figure 7–5) Simply by clicking on any item on the schedule, she can obtain more detail: a "patient at a glance" view of each scheduled patient, details concerning time and place of other engagements, etc. A counter box at the bottom of the screen keeps track of the time devoted to each encounter as input to the cost accounting system. As the day progresses, scheduled events are dropped from the display as each is completed. If during the day a patient telephones the practice to cancel an appointment or request an urgent, acute appointment, the Triage Nurse in the clinic or Dr. Livingston's secretary can schedule the encounter and the revised schedule is displayed immediately on Dr. Livingston's Care Station.

The workstation includes a number of action bars that provide quick access to information and assist Dr. Livingston in managing all of her communications with colleagues and patients. Across the very top of the display in Figure 7-5 are buttons that Dr. Livingston can use to access order entry and obtain lists and integrated results for any of her patients who have been admitted to an acute care or rehab hospital within the integrated delivery system. Other buttons provide access to tools that she may need to perform calculations or request analysis of data extracted from the database, access knowledge databases such as information about medications and toxic substances, and references such as

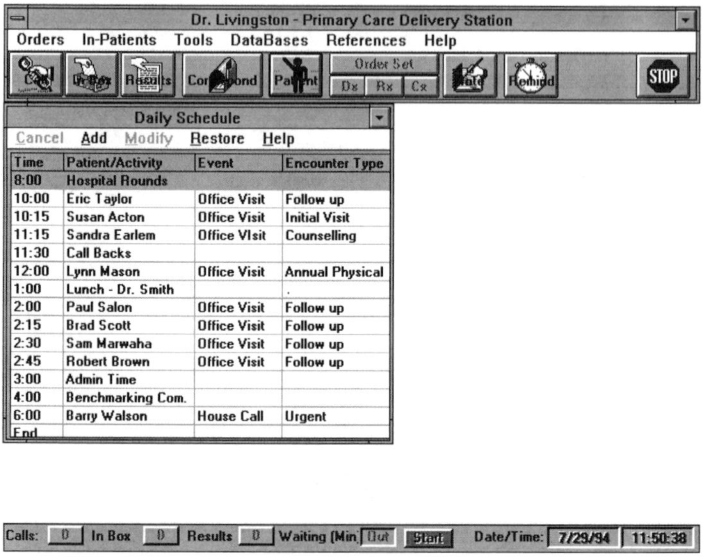

Figure 7-5. Role Visualization: Basic Display of Dr. Livingston's Care Station

the *Physician's Desk Reference,* clinical textbooks, or articles from the medical literature.

Across the next action bar are buttons Dr. Livingston is likely to use often during her work day. The Calls button allows her to review telephone messages logged in by staff in the clinic. She can store these online until she feels the inquiry has been managed to closure, and use the display as a template to document her response and any outcome for patient management that should be recorded in the patient's health history maintained in the system. The counter at the bottom of the workstation display keeps a running total of the new telephone messages and turns red to alert Dr. Livingston about any urgent calls.

Dr. Livingston is connected via electronic mail to all of her colleagues within the clinic and throughout the integrated care delivery system; she receives all administrative announcements and notifications from the Health Care Management Team electronically. She can review these, as well as any faxes received, by activating the In-Box button. A counter at the bottom of the screen displays the number of new electronic messages awaiting her review.

The Results button accesses the system application that assists Dr. Livingston in managing her review of and response to all diagnostic studies performed on patients in her panel. The counter at the bottom of the screen keeps a running total of new results posted, and, like the Calls button, turns red when stat or critical value results are added to her electronic results "in box."

The Correspondence button provides access to templates that Dr. Livingston uses to write school and camp letters, letters to patients concerning routine diagnostic and health screening results, and other correspondence to patients, payers, employers, and professional colleagues. She can incorporate any patient information from the system automatically and add free-text notes to any template via voice recognition. Completed correspondence can be mailed, faxed, or sent via electronic mail, depending upon the options available for each recipient.

The Patient button allows quick access to integrated views of patient information. Dr. Livingston can request views of patient data in many different slices through data types and time: Patient at a Glance, Visit at a Glance, Problem-Oriented, Chronological Series, Most Recent Results, Health Maintenance Status, etc.

The Order Set button calls up sets of orders and instructions based on clinical guidelines and care pathways that the Clinical Practice Management Team maintains on an ongoing basis. Dr. Livingston is notified of any updates/enhancements via electronic mail. (Her daily schedule in Figure 7-5 shows that she herself will be attending one of the regular meetings of the Benchmarking Subcommittee that monitors internal performance against standards). When specific protocols have been approved by a patient's payer, she is guided by the system in matching the patient with the preapproved care plan. Dr. Livingston can use the three buttons below Order Set, to place individual orders for diagnostic studies, prescriptions, or consultations.

Dr. Livingston activates the next button, Notes, when she needs to document a patient visit or telephone consultation. She can easily incorporate prescriptions, test orders and results, or any other information available in the system and enter her text note via keyboard entry, voice recognition, or a combination of these modes.

By activating the Remind button, Dr. Livingston can enter patient-specific reminders concerning follow-up. She can set these up for a future date for herself or for other members of the clinical team in her clinic. Each day, she reviews her "to dos" for the day.

Preparing for Hospital Rounds

The first item on Dr. Livingston's agenda today is checking on her patients who are currently hospitalized. After logging on to her Care Station, she accesses the Inpatients button and pulls down the menu to select a current patient listing, as shown in Figure 7-6. This displays which patients are currently in each hospital, along with their current location (inpatient unit, room, and bed) to aid Dr. Livingston in completing her rounds efficiently. She also calls up a preformatted rounds report listing all patient status information (vital signs, nurse charting against the clinical pathway, and notes for deviations from expected status) from the initial nursing assessment for the day and diagnostic results reported out within the last 24 hours. She loads all of this information into her Personal Digital Assistant (PDA), which she will take with her during her hospital rounds.

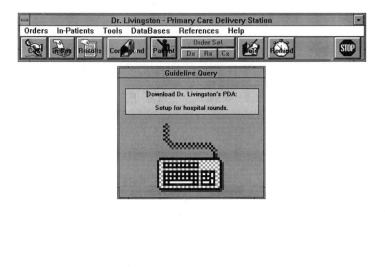

Figure 7-6. Role Visualization: Preparation for Hospital Rounds

During her rounds, Dr. Livingston will also be able to sign onto her personal workstation at terminals located in each inpatient unit to check for more current information, update care plans and patient information based on her assessment, and check for telephone and other messages that have been logged.

First Clinic Patient of the Day

When Dr. Livingston returns to the clinic, she sees her first patient, Eric Taylor. When she clicks on his entry in her daily schedule, the system pulls in a Patient at a Glance summary for Eric, as shown in Figure 7-7. Dr. Livingston has been following Eric for hypertension, and this visit was scheduled for a routine blood pressure check. The system is flagging (in red) a cholesterol reading for Eric that is above normal limits. This resulted from a health screening program that the Health Plan conducted at Eric's place of work since his last visit to Dr. Livingston.

Dr. Livingston first checks Eric's blood pressure, and, finding it still on the high side, tells Eric that she will be increasing his dosage of Procardia. To accomplish this she pulls down the menus under the Rx button and notes the change in dosage. The system automatically notifies the Pharmacy where Eric routinely picks up his medications so that the correct prescription is on file when he stops there later in the day.

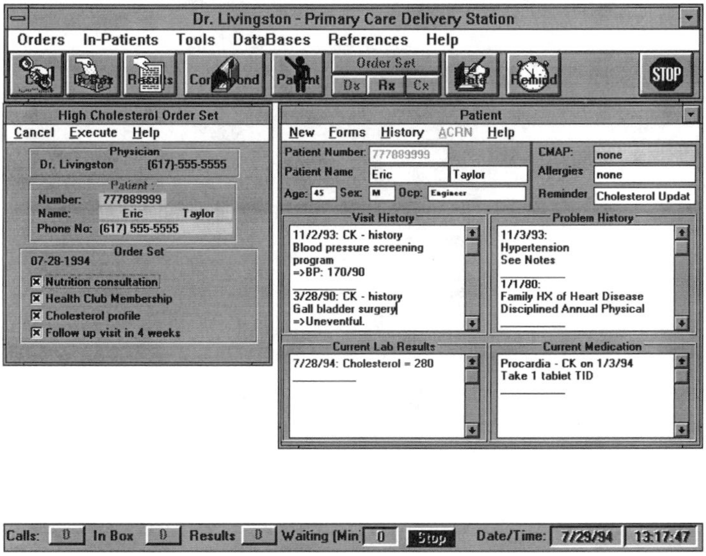

Figure 7-7. Role Visualization:Patient at a Glance and Protocol for Follow-up of Elevated Cholesterol

Now turning her attention to Eric's elevated cholesterol, Dr. Livingston accesses the protocol prenegotiated with Eric's insurance carrier, and activates each intervention as she discusses them with Eric (window in Figure 7-7). When she activates these items in the protocol, the system automatically notifies the Nutrition Clinic that Eric will be calling to schedule a consultation and the receptionist in her clinic to schedule another follow-up appointment for Eric in 4 weeks. Eric is eligible for a discount on a membership in a Health Club affiliated with the Health Plan; Dr. Livingston explains this to Eric and activates the item in the protocol, automatically notifying the Health Club via electronic mail that Eric has been approved for a discounted membership for medical reasons. She also orders a full cholesterol profile for Eric; he will need to make an appointment at the Health Office at his employer to draw a specimen in 3 weeks so the results will be available in time for his follow-up visit.

After explaining all of these interventions, Dr. Livingston downloads a set of complete instructions to Eric's PDA, as shown in Figure 7-8. The system has already determined the next available appointments for Eric in the Nutrition Clinic and in Dr. Livingston's clinic. He will need to call to confirm or change these.

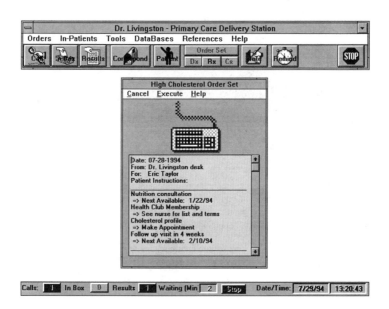

Figure 7-8. Role Visualization: Downloading of Patient Instructions to Patient's Personal Digital Assistant

Urgent Telephone Message

While Dr. Livingston has been seeing Eric, the Calls and Results counters at the bottom of the display on her Care Station have both turned red, and she decides to check these urgent messages before seeing her next patient. She clicks on the Calls button and the system brings up an urgent telephone message from a visiting nurse who is at the home of one of her patients, Paul Gates, as well as the Patient at a Glance view of this patient. The system automatically places the return telephone call at Dr. Livingston's prompt, and Dr. Livingston and the visiting nurse discuss the situation while Dr. Livingston views the display of the telephone message and data for Paul Gates on her workstation screen (Figure 7–9).

The visiting nurse made her routine call to check up on Dr. Gates, who is a retired physician with chronic pulmonary disease. She felt he was having difficulty breathing and performed a blood oximetry reading that confirmed her assessment. She transmitted this reading to the patient database (hence, the red alert on Dr. Livingston's Results counter and the corresponding entry in the Patient at a Glance display for Paul Gates).

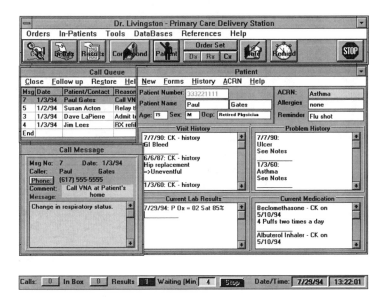

Figure 7-9. Role Visualization: Telephone Message from Visiting Nurse and Patient at a Glance for Patient Being Managed with Home Care

Dr. Livingston and the visiting nurse decide that Dr. Gates should be admitted for further evaluation and treatment. To accomplish this, Dr. Livingston pulls down the protocol (Figure 7-10) and checks off the appropriate interventions and notifications. The system will automatically notify the ambulance service of the patient's address, condition, and destination; discontinue home care services for Dr. Gates for the duration of his hospitalization; and notify the Pulmonary Team at the hospital to expect Dr. Gates' arrival and put him on the clinical pathway for acute exacerbation of asthma in adults. The display also reminds Dr. Livingston to notify other family members of her decision to admit this patient (Dr. Gates lives alone and his son is routinely notified).

Dr. Livingston sets a "to do" reminder for herself to check on Paul Gates at the conclusion of her morning clinic session and then turns her attention back to her clinic patients by clicking on the next patient displayed on her schedule. In this manner, Dr. Livingston routinely relies upon her Care Station as an indispensable information partner supporting her direct care role in the integrated care delivery system.

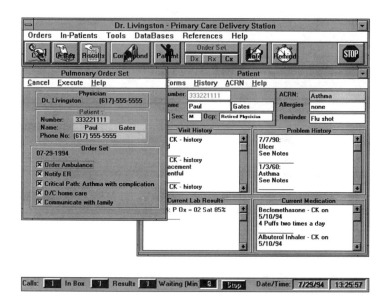

Figure 7-10. Role Visualization: Protocol for Admitting Adult Patient with Exacerbation of Asthma

References

1. Drazen E, Dietrich ʌ
   restructuring. Proceedirfoformation systems to support patient-focused
   Health Information Managhe Annual HIMSS Conference. Chicago, IL:
2. Institute of Medicine, Clinit Systems Society, 1994:1:229-238.
   Program, Washington, DC: Naactice Guidelines. Directions for a New
3. American Medical Association, ʟAcademy Press, 1990.
   Sources, and Updates, Chicago, IL: 'pry of Practice Parameters. Titles,
   Medical Review, 1993.   \ Office of Quality Assurance and
4. Gottlieb LK, Sokol HN, Murrey KO, et aι.
   improvement. Clinical guidelines and conorithm-based clinical quality
   HMO Practice 1992;6(1):5-12.   ous quality improvement.
5. Lumsdon K, Hagland M. Mapping care. Hospι ς & Health Networks
   1993;67(19):34-40.
6. O'Leary DS. The measurement mandate: Report \rd day is coming.
   Journal on Quality Improvement 1993;19:487-491.
7. Lawthers AG, Palmer RH, Edwards JE, et al. Developiι and evaluating
   performance measures for ambulatory care quality: a prelinγary report of
   the DEMPAQ Project. Journal on Quality Improvement 1993;ν552-565.
8. Bergman R. Making the grade. Report cards will be used to mιasure the
   performance of health plans: how might they work? Hospitals ᴄHealth
   Networks 1994;70(1):34-36.
9. National Council on Quality Assurance. Health Plan Employer Data αnd
   Information Set and Users' Manual, Version 2.0. NCQA, Washington, DC,
   1993.
10. Nerenz DR, Zajac BM, Rosman HS. Consortium research on indicators of
    system performance (CRISP). Journal on Quality Improvement 1993;19:577-
    585.
11. Nadzam DM, Turpin R, Hanold LS, et al. Data-driven performance
    improvement in health care. The Joint Commissions's Indicator
    Measurement System (IMSystem). Journal on Quality Improvement
    1993;19:492-500.
12. Anonymous. Full steam ahead! Survey confirms rush to join networks.
    Hospitals & Health Networks 1993;67(20):18.
13. Bergman R. A doctor in the network. Physician links improve access to
    critical data. Hospitals & Health Networks 1993;67(20):25-26.
14. Anonymous. The Evolution of a Community Network. Community
    Medical Network Society, November 1993.
15. Greco PJ, Eisenberg JM. Changing physicians' practices. New England
    Journal of Medicine 1993;329:1271-1274.
16. Drazen E, Metzger J, Stasior D. Letter to the Editor. New England Journal
    of Medicine 1994;330:436

17. Drazen E, Marwaha S. Outcomes: Who's M... What? Presentation at the College of Health Information Manag... Executives (CHIME) CIO Forum, Phoenix, AZ, February 1994.

18. Marwaha S. The role environment p... tive: Gearing technology to the needs of the business. Arthur D. Li... c. Connect, 1993;4(3)8-13.

Index